STALKING YANG

Finding Your Tai Chi Body

STALKING YANG LU-CHAN
Finding Your Tai Chi Body

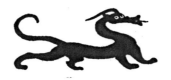

Robin Johnson

SUNSTONE
PRESS

SANTA FE

Sunstone books may be purchased for educational, business, or sales promotional use.
For information please write: Special Markets Department, Sunstone Press,
P.O. Box 2321, Santa Fe, New Mexico 87504-2321.

Library of Congress Cataloging-in-Publication Data:

Johnson, Robin, 1938-
    Stalking Yang Lu-Chan : finding your Tai chi body / by Robin Johnson.
        p. cm.
    ISBN 0-86534-482-5 (softcover : alk. paper)
    1. Tai chi. I. Title.

GV504.J66 2005
613.7'148—dc22

                                                    2005019600

Published in
Santa Fe

WWW.SUNSTONEPRESS.COM
SUNSTONE PRESS / POST OFFICE BOX 2321 / SANTA FE, NM 87504-2321 /USA
(505) 988-4418 / ORDERS ONLY (800) 243-5644 / FAX (505) 988-1025

For Rhiannon my daughter

CONTENTS

PREFACE

There are many books on Tai Chi Chuan, or at least Tai Chi, to be read, scanned, sampled, or placed back on the shelf. Most are interesting, in line with the Chinese suggestion that one may live in interesting times. Few address Tai Chi Chuan simply as a human generality, as Common Sense, which is what beginners and long-term students alike need to progress. They need practical guides. Scholars may prefer literature from high places. Poetry and calligraphy, though admirable and complex art forms, may not be the best mediums for everyday feet-on-the-ground learners And the old practice of secrecy in martial arts is just not tenable these days. Anyway, Tai Chi practice is in general very good for humans. It is also a dangerous art, as is archery, while being a peerless system of health-care. And Tai Chi Chuan is an absorbing sport and a richly intricate game.

Common ground for Tai Chi Chuan's uses is usually a solo form. This comprises relaxed flowing postures in a dance-like serial. Most practicers are learning or enacting a solo form, and most instruction is directed to this end. And by far the most common applications of Tai Chi form are general health and low-impact sport among two or more people. External practice is the best testing ground for Tai Chi skills. There are many competitions world-wide. Few of these can address Tai Chi Chuan's efficacy as a martial art in unstructured engagement. There are, however, many champions in specialized sporting forms, such as push-hands. More puzzling is competition in solo form, rather like a golf game without a ball.

Meanwhile, there seems to be a concern that standards are declining. With a huge and growing student body, the prospects are seated on a shaky foundation. Teachers will always appear to lead the throng, wherever it's headed. But no matter the standard, most of the work will be done solo. Well, isn't this where most is to be learned? From others maybe, but through you. Perhaps a decline makes less headway in a student remaining a student, than in one being led. What, after all, would the first Tai Chi student have done, in the absence of a teacher?

The methods proposed here address the principle underlying this question. Principles and secrets obscured by the smoke screen of classical literature are approached through own-body scrutiny. These methods aim also to enhance body-centered study of any form of extrinsic learning. And they have succeeded in effecting multiplied ability rather than fractional improvement. Self-learning and self-teaching can provide keys to doors revealing your body, your senses, your understanding; and, of course, your ignorance.

Propositions can be true or false. Your own body is the testing ground for these methods. Later, they may be applied and tested in partner-practice, eventually to any level of game. Once you have learned from yourself what these methods mean, they will have fulfilled their purpose, become redundant. Useful methods do take effort, as do useless ones, but the effort of hours or even minutes can yield dividends throughout your Tai Chi practice. In any event there is no bull in Tai Chi Chuan, your ability is soundly grounded in what you have done to acquire it.

THE FOUNDATION / WU JI
Stand up. Energy down
Tai Chi Chuan's fulcrum

Wu Ji is practiced widely as a solo standing exercise. It is a potent aid to healing diverse disharmony and sickness. How it works, while wholly unexplained, is likely linked to integration and self-repair. Humans seem to reap the benefits of sleep while standing upright and calmly alert.

Wu Ji could be described as standing for your life. It represents optimal economy in an upright person. Rather like cold immersion, Wu Ji standing directs attention to essential organs and processes. The exterior gets shunted to its more natural place, and the whole organism seems to get on better with life's main purpose.

Wu Ji standing by degrees inculcates a profound sense of internal integrity. Maintaining this integrity is a key to all subsequent Tai Chi movement. It's an expression of true economy, and is in effect Tai Chi Chuan's simplest posture.

Standing is not the only means to progress in Tai Chi Chuan; there are various spokes to the wheel. But Wu Ji is at the core of most methods: the hub of the wheel. Without its pivotal lessons, students will find it harder to sense the grace of essential movement, and their own intrinsic dimensions and conformation.

Initial efforts at acquiring many skills can, under Wu Ji's influence, condense to a singular practice. That is to maintain the deep internal integrity learned from standing; no more no less. The economy of Wu Ji's physical practice offers simple guidelines toward seamless movement. This is because still-standing alerts the stander to the noise of muddled intent. It is this noise which drowns out the subtle signals of a Wu Ji body. The quieter a body, the more sensitive it is to small energy or signals, whatever their source.

Wu Ji's energetics have been neatly illustrated by a TV ad for batteries. A powered toy keeps going after all others have run out of juice. The message here is that the most powerful battery wins. A Wu Ji take of the same event would be that the winner is the most energy-efficient toy. If there were 10 people standing for their lives, so to speak, all with identical and minimal resources, which one would be the last standing? The answer is not in the greatest power but in the greatest economy. This is a matter of not large, but small amounts of energy. The trend in Tai Chi practice is toward ever smaller amounts.

Since each person begins with the same resources or energy, how that energy is used is most important. By assigning minimal energy to the body's exterior, Wu Ji's aim, essential organs and functions may once more receive their due share. This essential balance of energies seems to generate Wu Ji's healing power. Persistent practice allows interior and exterior to use less and less energy as unneeded tensions inside and out are encouraged to release. Thus the organism integrates, as distinct from and opposed to the fragmentation that is sickness. Beneficial energy flows in the right amounts to the right places at the right times. Habitual divisions between organs, limbs, muscles, nerves, et al, melt away, and a more natural internal state prevails.

Initial practice may comprise various internal methods, such as diaphragm breathing, releasing muscles, generalizing the gaze, and centering limbs. Experience engenders a growing sense of internal uniformity, leading to a more singular application of attention. The former is many jobs, the latter tends toward one. Wu Ji standing can reduce the complexity of internal sensing to zero. Instinct or accumulated intelligence prevails over intellect, which is redundant in vital processes.

This outline of Wu Ji energetics suggests the difficulty of knowingly changing what has developed throughout one's lifetime. Habitual patterns of energy-use can be deep-rooted and far from the scrutiny of casual attention. That is why first approaches to Wu Ji tend to be more fruitful as a physical or structural exercise. How can someone address energy, especially excess energy, they may not know they're using? Habits often have obscure and forgotten origins. And efforts to get rid of unproductive ones can engender not less energy, but more, as one tension is exchanged for another.

As the body-mind, the organism, readjusts, signs may well manifest, such as twitching, tingling, numbness, coldness, or warmth. These in a way emanate from where instinct, body, and thinking-mind overlap. Such signs are just that; they will pass. Over-focusing on getting the posture right or even on merely standing for the first time can lead to dizziness. The first rule for all standing postures, and for self-defense, is don't forget to breathe. Sometimes just the thought of doing something difficult will induce a hardening of the abdomen and a virtual halt to respiration. The answer here and in general is to soften the body and let the diaphragm move downward.

In general, it's good practice to ease into Wu Ji standing. While adepts may stand for, say, an hour or two, starters will be better served with a few minutes. Thus trying Wu Ji several times a day will highlight the process of finding its structure. Then as clarity and confidence build, longer terms will no doubt ensue. Good instincts should be followed, and if in doubt take a break.

Physical tension can be located and released from most places in the body. Mental and emotional bad habits are less palpable and often more elusive. But they too can be let go. Calm nasal breathing is one method.

Paying excess attention to emotional and nervous quirks is a trap. It's just another way of holding on to them. Old habits are really good at what they do. But they are rather like food stains on a new shirt: you don't notice them arriving yet they tenaciously resist removal and displacement.

One's scrutiny of Wu Ji's processes should be neither too demanding nor too intense. Force is neither required nor desirable. Calm persistence and a cool attitude will bring all signs to pass. Many thousands have derived only good from Wu Ji standing.

As for the intellect, a quiet thinking-mind seems to act as a magnet for habits and detritus of excess thinking. These, too, may appear; they are stumbling blocks. Hapkido instructor Yoo Jun-saeng, once observed dryly that, no matter what you think, it's only in the mind. In other words, closed minds are good containers, whereas what may be needed is more openness in both thinking-mind and body. As usual, it was better advice than I realized at the time.

Wu Ji's standing structure is the physical vehicle for reducing noise, and opening the body and one's awareness of it. Wu Ji is in effect a high horse-stance with equal leg weighting but no flexure at the knees. Arms are fully pendent. Assembling body-components into Wu Ji structure may be better approached from the ground. Humans learn to stand from the head downward, allowing a floating head to indicate an optimal alignment with gravity. This process is initially instinctual. Adults usually have a far from instinctual sense of themselves, however. It seems better to begin assembling the body into its natural structure from the ground up, starting with the foot-soles.

Here are three ways of saying the same thing about placing the feet. First, the feet may be positioned merely by centering the hip joints, rather as a ball would center itself in a slightly larger bowl. Second, the legs should be self-centered and slightly pyramidal, not parallel. Third, the feet are placed under the shoulders, rather than directly under the pelvis.

In this latter alignment the thigh-bones will slope inward from hips to knees; not a stable set-up. In any case, foot-soles are sensed as flat on the ground with even weighting side-to-side and heel-pad-to-toe-pad (Chapter 2). Thus the center-lines of the feet will be parallel as if on tram lines. Most people will feel that their heels are overly separated. One reason for this is that many walk with their heels pulled inward or with the front of the feet splayed relative to each other. This habit is civilized and usually combines lower-back contraction with hip-joints collapsed backward.

Knees are at their maximum natural height from the ground; they rest just forward of locked. This unique position reflects centered knee joints, a position within which they easily wobble fore and back. The resulting arch from foot through pelvis to foot is stable, strong, and economical. I imagine it would stand even if, perhaps especially if, all flesh disappeared suddenly from the bones. The pelvis itself is slung, a state in which the sacrum, the hard triangular plate at the base of the spine, is vertical.

Again, a vertical sacrum may feel as if it needs to be held in position. Most modern humans sustain an outward-curved lower spine, from contraction and collapse. Some will have acquired an under-slung pelvis, this from frontal contraction and collapsed lower back. Whatever the problem, adopt a pelvic girdle that is relaxed between pushed back and pulled under. It's a structure that argues with locked knees. Locked knees are not relaxed, but collapsed, a position which allows force to dwell within the knee-joints. This stressed position is also immobilizing.

The modern militaristic practice of pulling shoulders up and back is reversed by relaxing the chest and softening the abdomen. Although this procedure is commonly described as sinking the chest, it is important to sink nothing; merely stop holding it up. Therefore one needs to let down an upwardly-contracted chest, and to complete the process by releasing any tightness between the shoulder-blades. This latter opening movement is often described as raising the back. Raise nothing; do not push or lift the upper back. Its natural outward curve reflects an absence of contraction or tension, which manifests as concavity centered on the spinal axis.

A main benefit of these adjustments is a more open spinal axis. The lower back is not collapsed inward, the upper spine is not forced outward. Smoothing the spine is completed by floating the head, placing its crown point on top. Floating the head also releases contraction at the back of the neck, a tension adopted by keeping the head up straight, so to speak. The admonition to hold the head as if suspended from above only seems to compound the problem of habitually tipped-back heads. Hold nothing; merely float the head on its synovial fluid. Small universal movements of the head will more or less locate the focus of this floating, where skull joins spine.

The structure within Wu Ji yields a person at his or her tallest while being optimally relaxed downward. Standing in this general state eventually opens up the interior to general scrutiny. No further practice is needed when this scrutiny of your inner structure actually reveals no divisions, no structure, so to speak. A sense of a you-shaped elastic outer membrane enclosing a uniform fluid may emerge. It did for me.

The following outline offers guidelines into Wu Ji's structure. Arriving at Wu Ji necessitates realizing and releasing habits of sustained tension throughout the organism, the body-mind. The basic method involves bringing attention to various parts of the organism. Attention is distinct from consciousness, thinking-mind, and gaze. The product of attention is awareness. Wu Ji standing is in part a process de-emphasizing the conscious hemisphere.

Bringing attention to the foot-soles encourages downward movement of tension, which is held or stuck energy. This general benefit is augmented by relaxing the feet including the foot-soles themselves. There can be a sense here of the ground soaking up into the feet as tension slips away.

At the same time it's important to let the body down into the feet. In other words letting the legs go a little will offer a more open path to downward energy. The feet may begin to feel more weight. In any case, weight within each foot and between both feet is even front-to-back and side-to-side (Chapter 2).

Get to know the feeling of heel- and toe-pads sitting evenly on the ground, something that may elude feet encased in modern trainers or shoes with even a small heel. If the toes are neither pulled up or back nor curled under, energy can flow to all parts of the feet. Minor changes in balance are bound to occur during extended standing. These can be readily sensed and compensated merely by maintaining even foot-soles. Sensing one's body as an internal practice is for most people an acquired or regained skill. A spirit of benevolent enquiry, enlightened self-interest, is a valuable asset in this quest.

Most energy entering Wu Ji feet comes from above and passes through the center of the ankles. When asked to indicate an ankle most people point to one or other of the protruding bones. The request is a trick. You must use both hands to encircle an ankle. (A similar scenario arises for knees, which are usually construed as the knee-caps) When weight is centered in the ankles they can become more relaxed. Sensing relaxed ankles is especially tricky because they are such dense joints, basically bone and cartilage. Try to collect experience from places in the body that you can willfully relax. Then apply the same approach to ankles. If you intend them to relax, eventually they will. Patience.

Knees, as distinct from ankles, are pure hinges. By centering the weight through this hinge the knee-caps can be encouraged to settle. Try locking knees, then releasing them forward, not downward, so that they quiver easily front-to-back. Many knees are habitually stressed side-to-side, unknown to their owners. Forceful and unnecessary thrusting, and collapse, are common conspirators in this abuse. Therefore, centering downward energy in knees can be a trying process, simple though it is.

Hip-joints are massive compared with knees and ankles. How can one sense the bony components and the degree of relaxation in supporting tissues? Not only are the joints deep, they are anchored from deeper within the lower torso. Nonetheless, laying a good foundation through feet, ankles, and knees can give some indication of a structure to learn. Softening the whole pelvic girdle will at least engender sympathetic relaxing in the hips. Repeated checking upward and downward, first for alignment, will make it easier to release. The more often one engages and reads the process, the more skilful interpretation becomes. A slightly floppy feel is a good counter to hardness and tension. Keep trying: you are relearning how you felt as an infant.

In any case, slightly pyramidal thighs should sit on knees, shanks, and feet rather like good plumbing would join tubes of slightly different diameters. There is a clear stability inherent in Wu Ji legs joined with a relaxed pelvis. You can feel it. It's a long-term arch, as standing can show. It's also a protoplasmic arch, which can be adjusted and tested for structure and efficiency each time you adopt Wu Ji.

Feet and legs too close can push ground energy up into the torso's center-line. Too wide tends to drag the body downward, splitting energy away from the center. Splayed feet, with fronts further apart than backs, will direct force into the lower back, where it will tend to collect. Learning these feelings is a challenge, and a door to progress.

It is unlikely that hips are well-set when the pelvis itself is not true to gravity. The sacrum is vertical in Wu Ji. Contracting the lower back to raise the tail, and the lower abdomen to draw it between the legs, offers brackets to the sacrum's central, vertical resting place. A relaxed sacrum has the feeling of being slung from the hips' ball-and-sockets. It is also the key to viable movement. A neutral sacrum allows the spinal axis to lengthen downward yielding a less concave lower back. This will lead to a more open connection with the thighs; the whole structure is smoother.

A similar concavity between shoulder-blades, engendered by an habitual shoulders-back attitude, is countered by letting the shoulders hit bottom, so to speak. They should sit on the top of the torso. Seen from above, natural shoulders form a curve whose center is somewhere in front of the body. Squared shoulders and a raised chest, enshrined in chest-out-shoulders-back, also cause tension in the upper-front torso. This is released by simply letting the chest down. A puffed-out chest is not viable, nor is it strong, despite its dogmatic appearance. In fact, it invades the diaphragm's downward action during inhalation. A tense back and front in the upper torso virtually severs above from below. This leads to a feeling of breath stuck at the level of the diaphragm. Perhaps this is because the diaphragm is out of practice.

A more open upper-torso lets the spine smooth out, allowing it to better connect and conduct. This is completed by floating the head. A head held up and back by contracting rear-neck muscles is another foible in modern deportment. Such an attitude directs vision horizontally. The human body is not a ram-rod: it curves slightly forward, rather like a bulldozer-blade. A floating head allows its internal balance-sensors to adopt their natural attitude. Relaxed general vision tends downward, meeting the ground a few body-lengths ahead. This is a much more realistic destination than a horizon that is always receding.

Small universal movements of the head indicate the head's fulcrum. Avoid large changes, especially exercises that force the head from its essentially vertical axis. Try to relax this inner fulcrum, and the muscles at the back of the neck. Even the thought of engaging in something effortful can induce tightening in the neck. So can stress and anger. A balanced head, relaxed torso, slung sacrum, and centered legs offer a smooth and flexible vertical axis through the body.

Arms are allowed to dangle, pendent (as in totally pendent) from the shoulders-joints. The upper-arms are rotated such that palms face backward. Lower-arms are not rotated at the elbows. This move aligns the arm foundations with the forward curve of the shoulder-shoulder line. Flow can now optimize between torso and vertical inactive arms. An externally active structure is what Wu Ji is not. So the upper-arm linkages need only to allow optimal internal flow during standing. (Arms seldom dwell in the vertical, or horizontal, during active engagement) Hands rest on the lateral apices of the outer thighs.

Downward energy passes through the foot-centers. These are aligned with the body's center of gravity, the perineum, and the crown point of the head. Feeling only its own weight, the head is buoyant compared with the rest of the body. Maintaining a floating head is one of the keys to effective engagement.

The preceding description of Wu Ji is summed up in standing naturally erect using the least energy possible. Then energy balances in favor of the vital interior, the source of all the rest, including thinking. Many everyday activities tend to favor the exterior **at the expense** of the interior vital organs. Reversing this pernicious relationship allows the general to direct the particular. And the body-mind moves toward its natural state of homeostasis and dynamic balance. De-emphasizing the exterior also leads to a quieter thinking-mind, in other words, the exterior-mind. And the neurological system quiets in a vertical but resting body, enhancing calmness and reducing stress.

Thus quieting either body or thinking-mind lessens the difference between them. Decisions are made lower in the body, guided by internal awareness. It is more a process of the thinking-mind melding with the body, than the converse.

Although the foregoing may suggest otherwise, Wu Ji is not a matter of words. But it **is** a matter of breathing. The breath is the heart of Wu Ji. It is a simple matter. Air entering the nose is allowed to fall toward the body's center. There is no interference from the rib-bellows. Inhaling is adding fluid to a fluid-filled, human-shaped membrane. Inhalation induces this elastic membrane, our outer layers, to radiate outward from the center or lower dantien. A sensitive scale would reveal a weight increase. At the same time the whole body would become less dense with greater volume. This is a comfortable unforced expansion.

Exhalation begins as diaphragm and rib-muscles reach a limit of elastic contraction. Letting breath out through the nose induces a steady condensing or spherical shrinking of the body, which includes limbs. The periphery falls and flows toward the center. Diaphragm and rib muscles release into an elastic limit. Then the next breath cycle begins.

The breath-rate tends to slow during Wu Ji: increased relaxation, less interference, and less need for air. Breathing may become deeper and softer. Rhythms smooth and move toward the center. Vital internal organs enjoy enhanced relationships. A sense of difference or fragmentation fades. There is a cool feel that persists even in the heat of engagement; one view of stillness in motion.

Hands are the ends of Wu Ji's fully pendent arms. A long history of tool-use imbues humans with a sense of hands as a center And less usefully, as a body's leader, to be followed regardless of that body's intrinsic functions. Tai Chi practice makes full use of the hands' appropriate abilities. But in the same way Tai Chi-hands are used as if they were the ends of the arms. Who would argue with this? And as such, hands should express the general form of the parent arms. In other words, a hand's profile should present a shallow curve. This curve is compound, radiating from a hand's center, whose location lies on a projection of a fore-arm's core.

With the butt at the hair-line, a Tai Chi-hand fits easily over its owner's cranium. This is not the shape of most peoples' relaxed, open hands. Most hands reflect habitual contraction with fingers hooked inward as if carrying something. Opening hands to their natural curve needs effort, to adopt, and to remember. Circulation through the arms, aided by rotation of the upper-arms, can now flow unimpeded to the ends of all digits.

Wrists are straight such that the fore-arm cores project along the center digits. Structure from shoulder to finger-tips is smooth; function can move seamlessly throughout an arm. And there is no need to prepare a hand for action: it is already in shape, even for percussive use of finger-tips.

Wu Ji-hands also offer a common-sentient analog of overall bodily structure. Each has a more massive core from which radiate five appendages. One of these is a little different from the other four. One can relate torso/palm, limbs/fingers, and head/thumb. Tai Chi-body and -hand present similar curvature, a function of a similar centering. The digits of a natural hand unfold outward from the palm-center. This is located along the arm's core-line where it passes through the base or butt of the palm. Eventually this slight curve or Tai Chi-straight is maintained without conscious attention, as in the so-called turtle-back of the torso.

Wu Ji-standing with fully pendent arms presents considerable fluid pressure in the hands. A result is fingers like those of a fluid-filled rubber glove. The thumbs are allowed to flatten against the thighs' outer mid-lines, but without folding the smooth curve between thumbs and index fingers (tiger-mouth). Hands thus remain fully connected internally despite the arms being inactive externally. Elbows sit out slightly from the torso, a structure maintained in all Tai Chi practice. Elbows are not lifted one iota; the arms are fully pendent.

Experts differ on placing the tongue-tip. The issue is putative pathways of internal energy-flow. It may be that a particular position suits an adopted or artificial technique of specialization, such as sitting meditation, or energy management. Are such special arrangements congruent with a natural body's generality? No one has proven any best technique, or even a necessity for this practice. Experts do tend to be specialists.

However, practice dwells in three positions. First, no special placement; second, the tongue-tip adheres to the upper palate adjacent to the center incisors; third, adhering to the upper palate during inhalation and lying down during exhalation. Whatever works in the long term without side-effects is no doubt suitable. Tai Chi principles would suggest the least contrived method. In any case, what matters most is that the Wu Ji posture is in place, and breathing has a natural un-forced rhythm.

Each person's unique structure offers a singular approach to Wu Ji. Adopting Wu Ji is a process of releasing unproductive tension or contraction, a matter of both energy and substance. Releasing can be easy in, say, fingers, and difficult in hips and ankles. A dense joint like an ankle is mostly bone and sinew: how does one release gristle? And hips, large and complex, are buried deep, far from easy scrutiny.

But persistence works. The will that beats your heart is persistent is it not? Repeated relaxing downward, softening bulk muscle, yields a softer body, and reveals its intrinsic elasticity. Excess energy finds its way out of the body via relaxed foot-soles or digit-tips of open hands. Progress brings awareness of stuck energy in places and at levels initially hidden among the noise of general tension. Tai Chi Chuan's peerless efficacy as a martial art is seated in its effortless management of minimal energy. Eventually, this awareness helps release any stagnant mass and energy within your body, and engenders a sense of powerful well-being.

Progress to all levels is assured by common sense, a good attitude, and benevolent patience. Anxieties about mental and emotional rebalancing will melt away. You can always talk with a more experienced student, or simply go for a walk. The apparent complications of initial practice may invite ill-informed intensity. Relax. The aim is to be comfortable. Not getting something right in your approach to the complexity of your natural body is not a cause for complaint. Competence emerges from basics applied at every level.

Wu Ji's power to integrate and cure is founded in the body-mind's awareness of imbalances when small or emerging. Whatever the explanation, Wu Ji is attractively simple: stand up and let go.

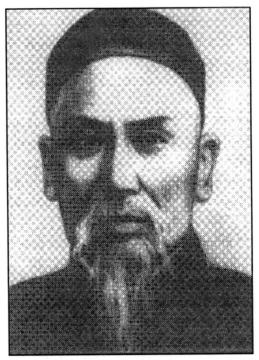

Yang Lu-chan (1799–1872 A.D.)

INTRODUCTION
Presenting the student
(Teacher included)

Perhaps he was lucky as well as astute. The oft-told story of Yang Lu-chan's nightly vigils at the Chen-family village in Henan province began with a chance. He stumbled on the vista of Chen students practicing secretly after dark. No doubt unaware of it, he applied a basic Tai Chi tactic: he seized the opportunity; he watched. And then, following another important principal, he persevered, both in his vigils, and in his own practice of what he felt he saw.

This tale may be factual or even allegory for Tai Chi principles, or some of each. Whatever the origin, stories such as this exist because they are useful. It certainly serves as a fitting opening stanza in an epic saga of Tai Chi Chuan.

The story continues with Yang progressing so well, without oral instruction, that his skills prevailed over others' in the class. And his hard work, solo work, and persistence, brought the Chen family's respect and direct instruction in the complete art.

Today, many thousands clearly benefit from this hazy aspect of Yang-family history. But I want to go back to that first verse, when there was just one person forced to learn alone. Yang Lu-chan did well what we all have to do to some degree: learn from oneself; become student **and teacher.** This, for me , renders redundant the precise details of this piece of history. Rather, it puts me in Yang's shoes, asking first, "How should it feel to do what I saw?" And then, "Exactly?"

These two questions arose from a situation similar to Yang's. I had two chances annually to observe the Yang-style short form performed by Prof. Cheng Man-ching. Between viewings, I could only try again and again to re-enact memories of someone else's moves; Tai Chi groups were rare in those days. And even if you now enjoy direct teaching, you still have to practice many times what you might have seen only a few.

Several hours of daily practice had its (modest) rewards for me, as it did (royally) for Yang Lu-chan. Like the proverbial monkey at the typewriter, I stumbled on orders and rhythms through sheer mind-numbing repetition. Forming my body over and over to mnemonic replays of just one or two moves, eventually brought some sense of core principles. Every Tai Chi practicer will know that I couldn't be sure of what I was learning. I could only iterate and reiterate: release, align, and sink. And trust blindly in my emerging instincts.

Why, though, should self-teaching interest today's students, for whom texts, videos, and those wishing to teach abound? One reason is precisely because any serious student of internal arts can receive only guidelines and inspiration from teachers or demonstrations. Most of the work is done within, as we try to put details of our solo efforts into the context of Tai Chi general principles.

Small successes bridge the gap a little. And because Tai Chi Chuan is an integrated art, any realized connection becomes a valuable learning device or analog: a hint at the general. In effect, one approaches in action the kind of principle expounded in Classic aphorisms. This is no small achievement, although you may believe otherwise at the time. Learning to realize the Classics in practice must surely be important to serious students (as is realizing how obscure those texts can be).

Equally important, repetition (itself a "hidden" technique; elusive because it isn't done enough) is almost certain to reveal structure to questing scrutiny. And structure gives form to the "details," as do the rules of plant growth to the mind-boggling structure of leaves on a tree. I am sure this concept is behind teachers saying, "Again, please," a hundred times (or "Again, please, a hundred times," depending on the student). Progress in Tai Chi Chuan seems to depend on practicing a few things a thousand times, rather than the converse.

In the realm of self-teaching, just how I conducted these few things evolved as core devices in a personal training manual of internal practice. A similar process unfolds now as I learn to use my hands, first with single digits, then as various combinations, and first consciously, then internally. This approach has yielded methods that have withstood more than three decades of application and skeptical scrutiny. And applied by many students, they have served well in my aim to render my function as an instructor redundant. They are:

1. Never forget Wu Ji.
2. The center-line.
3. Hinging and rotation.
4. To raise the toe…
5. Similar limbs.
6. Sling the rear knee.
7. Horse-stance method.
8. Misreading orientation.
9. Powers of ten.
10. Perfect balance.

The essence of these guidelines can be apprehended in just a few steps of form (in any style, if there is such in functional Tai Chi Chuan), plus Wu Ji standing, and Opening (in my case, of the Cheng short form).

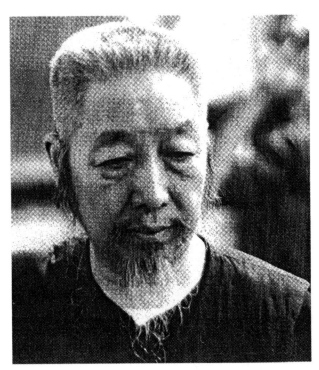

Cheng Man-ching (1901–1975 A.D.)

1

NEVER FORGET WU JI
Moving inside out
Still fluid dynamics

Forget the thinking-mind instead. This is the very practical matter of preserving Wu Ji integrity throughout the body dynamics of each move. It is recalling while moving, physical impressions learned from standing still. Imprinting these recollections into a moving body requires experience. No amount of thinking or theory will do. For some, this may take a few hours of practice; for most of us, many hours. The repertoire of a Tai Chi form in all its variety of steps and combinations is a demanding engagement. Perhaps more daunting are tenacious habits of deportment and movement imbued by specious demands of modern, civilized life.

Meanwhile, such things as a floating head, suspended (vertical) sacrum, and open hands are a few learned impressions that you can apply directly by feel. It can help to let your attention, that is, relaxed scrutiny, dwell on just one sensation in Wu Ji, then to take that impression into subsequent movements. One reason why this is so useful is that memory leaves the thinking-mind and seeps into the body, then begins to transform into instinct. Thus consciousness quiets, leading to less noise and therefore clearer signals.

Remembering Wu Ji is especially useful for melting tension and letting go. Each of these reverses formidable habits. You can stop moving anytime and patiently apply Wu Ji relaxation. For example, just what do Wu Ji's completely pendent, tensionless arms feel like? Then resume moving after recognizing some improvement in feel. Maintaining proper relaxation into your first posture, whatever it is, is a key to the whole form. Releasing counter-productive tension and reducing neurological noise are real steps toward the principle of stillness within motion.

Wu Ji is an effective medium through which to relate experience in one region of the body to another. We have four limbs, which in our usual upright posture, are oriented downward. The arms are pendent, thus extended, and the legs, which bear our weight, are compressed. It can be relatively easy to release the arms, to let go, because they can be allowed to hang. If you are standing reasonably well, arms can be sensed as a whole, realizing their intrinsic structure. By which I mean, organs are self-aware; they know when they're in one piece, so to speak. Arms are, after all, organs of manipulation and locomotion. Conscious release of tension in arms can lead to sensing them as a whole: their shape from the inside, and their energetic state and configuration. So hanging arms are one possible key to both form and emptiness.

Getting to know just what an arm or any region feels like needs time. However well the idea seats, or makes sense, it is essential to give yourself enough time to learn what the experience is through body-senses. It may take an hour or many to become familiar with this unusual approach to what you are doing. But experience counts. It's very helpful in early stages to return to a simple exercise like feeling out the hanging arms. The process is internal, like eyes looking down an arm as they would a tunnel. In this case it is inner vision or feeling. With practice, which means repetition, what it is you are trying to do will be clearer. Then you can begin applying your new-found experience as a tool. The ability multiplies with each new scenario. But give yourself time. Arms, being suspended, are relatively accessible.

Legs, which are compressed most of the time, are more difficult. These, too, are organs of locomotion and manipulation, but their size relative to arms hints at both more energy and more substance to deal with when trying to let go. The one-sense that I've referred to in the arms can be directly applied to achieving the same in the legs. You are, after all, retrieving a sense or feel of something that's already happened, albeit elsewhere. That is one of the very useful experiences I gained from Wu Ji standing. If I could get my compressed legs to feel as relaxed as my suspended arms, I would be making progress. And I find that this kind of intra-body communication can be very useful in itself and in the overall process of full integration.

The structure of a Wu Ji arm is also a sure guide to viable structure in movement. A slightly curved pendent arm, arcing from shoulder to fingertips, is a fully open structure. It's a curved tube, a flexible conduit for ready flow of intrinsic energy. Engaging the Opening process at the form's beginning expresses a pendent arm-sense transforming into a rising (that is, moving) arm-sense while leaving the elbows exactly as they were when hanging. Wrists are at shoulder-joint height; no higher. Elbows have not flexed one iota. You have now moved a Wu Ji arm merely by using the shoulder-joint. Meanwhile, one can sense the arms' weight along their undersides. With repeated relaxation and letting go, as in Wu Ji, eventually they will rise from vertical to horizontal with "no" physical effort. Also, horizontal arms eventually feel almost like vertical ones, yielding maximum internal openness allowed by the structure. Furthermore, such a change expresses the essence of most arm movements throughout the form (There is a different pattern of energy employed when an elbow moves above the shoulder-joint), offering a powerful tool for achieving effortless movement throughout the body.

The next change to the arms is flexing the elbows. Continuing the sequence of Opening, this requires letting the elbows fall to their lowest natural position. This is in line with the torso's lateral vertical axis which runs from the shoulder joint, under the armpit, and down through the hip joint, on each side of the body. If the arms move any further, the elbows will begin to rise backward: a different kind of energy. The constraint of maintaining hands at the same separation throughout Opening will also cause the elbows to move out from the torso. That is, something rises without being lifted (which I consider to be an important principle in Tai Chi movement; lift nothing. Arms, legs, and their parts rise because energy is moving **along** them). The main question now is, "How much should they flex?"

Well, so that the elbow-joint is more open than closed. This, like all other bodily forms, can be sensed. In modern, civilized bodies this might take considerable self-training. However, an elbow that is flexed more than about 90 degrees will have passed this crucial position. The real meaning of an elbow more open than closed is a fully functional arm. That is, any part of it can be applied to any Tai Chi technique without requiring force. Can the fingertips still express piercing energy (rooted in the feet, of course)? Can the arm be maintained without physical force when attacked from any direction? Testing will answer these and other questions about a Tai Chi-fully flexed elbow.

Clearly, one can empty any part of the body, elbows and wrists included. We just need to be aware of this; it is something we intend to do. In other words, when the wrist is empty (something quite apparent in Cheng's arms during Opening) the hands are energetically redundant. Similarly, a fully-folded elbow isolates the arm below it from active engagement (a common move in the technique of folding). The guiding principle in elbow and other joint flexing is whether or not that joint is rounded, as distinct from angled. This is less a matter of external scrutiny and more one of internal sensing.

The movements of Opening thus set up the parameters for long and short arms, and by analogy, the legs, and even the body as a whole. For example, the next structure, Hold-the-ball (which is not holding a ball), comprises a long or pendent lower arm plus a folded upper arm, each with its hand-center aligned with the nose-navel line. It bears repeating that shoulders remain open. The upper arm is horizontal, the wrist level with the shoulder, but with the elbow settled but not sunk. The palm faces down. As for the lower arm, its sits at the other end of the torso, with the palm rotated upward (but not horizontal; the wrist is Tai Chi-straight). In other words, it's the same-shaped arm as the one that floated upwards in Opening, except that it is also gently curved to bring the palm-center to the nose-navel line.

And the principles move on through the form, illuminating all subsequent structures. Wu Ji standing is really the source of not only seamless structure but also optimal economy (Is there any other kind?) for all Tai Chi form and movement. Repetition and application are the training methods for approaching these intrinsic skills.

2

THE CENTER-LINE
Knees wave like flags
Soles at one with the ground

Maintaining equal weight in both sides of a line dividing each foot lengthwise has proved to be very simple and very useful. Observing the center-line applies to standing, movement, feet on or off the ground, and at any speed.

The line joins the working center of each heel-pad ("heel") and toe-pad ("toe") within each foot. These pads are described commonly as balls, which they are not. Balls are round, whereas these pads are essentially flat. Their properties can be ascertained readily by conducting a slow spin on each. Note that lifting the front or back of a foot prior to testing its pads will lift part of the pad from the ground (Chapter 4).

It doesn't help to look at a foot's exterior form; the center-line is at floor-level. It is actually slightly curved. But parallel-footed, for example, means that the distance between feet is the same heel-to-heel and toe-to-toe (Note the above definitions).

Feet evenly flat (How else can they be flat?) on the ground is fundamental to Tai Chi practice. A foot-sole is not intrinsically flat, of course, but weight from above should be distributed as if it were. As practice advances, more of your foot-soles will reach the ground. Letting the feet rock from side to side is surely a sign of basic instability. Observing the center-line is simply a corollary of conducting energy through the center of the limbs above, a natural attribute of a natural body. And basic locomotion comprises energy moving along the center-line, whether the energy is entering or leaving.

Postures and steps in solo form eventually feel so much more stable, therefore relaxed, when foot-soles are congruent with the floor. Very slow movement is very good for both observing the center-line and programming the body-memory. Another general test of the center-line's efficacy is partner practice at a slow enough pace to sense the changing dynamics in the foot-soles.

Sinking and rising in a horse-stance is a specific structure within which to test center-line maintenance. It is easy to let weight drift to one side of the feet or one foot as the knees flex and straighten. It may not be so easy to detect it, however. One reason is that transverse rolling of the feet is common in modern locomotion. Thus it may be difficult to sense as impractical, something that one usually does. Rather than analyze each person's idiosyncrasies, it may simply be better to place foot-soles flat on the ground.

Again, very slow sinking and rising allows real-time corrections of any sidedness that may manifest. Initial placing of feet under the shoulders, that is, adopting slightly pyramidal legs, and orienting them along parallel lines is crucial. Maintaining the center of gravity, the lower dantien, midway between the feet helps the sense of identical foot-soles on the ground. This internal scrutiny by the mover can be matched with leg alignment as seen by a partner, or in a mirror.

Knees act like flags. Even a slight wobble at floor level is readily discerned higher up the leg. It is better than otherwise to accept **no** leeway in centering knee joints; energy must pass through the core of the main joint.

The next consideration is sensing the center-lines of heavy and light feet. A relatively high horse-stance is a good place to begin this exploration. Since the weight is centered, it's necessary to shift torso-weight to one leg, and that means one leg only. The other leg will need to be as fully pendent, hanging from the hip, as the position allows. Without first lowering the center, you'll note that it's virtually impossible to place and feel the lighter, torso-empty foot-sole flat on the ground. Well, you can do it if you sway the pelvis, which will cause the lighter side to dip. That, of course, is counter to Tai Chi strategy; it's not some detail. (You may sway the pelvis because you need to according to unfolding circumstances, as in combat, but that's another matter: you know what you are doing)

So the center needs to be low enough to enable shifting a plumb pelvic girdle over one leg **without one iota of thrust from the emptying leg**. If the leg is thrusting, how can it possibly be emptying? Another way to approach this fully-differentiated structure is to lower the center into one leg with a clear sense of the light leg just hanging. Move it floppily just to make sure. Then flop it into position about a shoulder-width from the other leg with the feet parallel. If you have lowered enough, the sole of the empty foot will sit flat on the ground, which means with the weight even on each side of its center-line. Test this weighted-ness until you're absolutely sure of evenness. Bring the attention back to the standing leg (the torso-full one), and make sure that it too is centered. Check the pelvis. Then as an exercise, do the best to flop an empty foot within the structural parameters you have just set up, not once, but many times.

The word empty is a relative term denoting a foot on the ground free of torso-weight. To feel a truly empty limb, stand on a step or other raised surface that will allow one limb to hang while you stand on the other. (I use a nine-inch block, big enough for one foot) The full weight of the hanging leg can now be sensed at the pelvic joint. It is worth getting to know this feeling, because it is to leg movement what Wu Ji-feel is to movement in general. Even when a leg is allowed to hang onto the ground, it is not quite the same as when it is hanging in the air. And when merely stepping, the "empty" leg is imbued with some action, that is, muscle-use. It is therefore not quite empty, and is sensed as such with adequate practice. But you can feel that most of its energy is downward. Persevere because civilized bodies and natural bodies are virtual distant relatives.

Maintaining the center-line in flying legs, especially at slow speeds, needs close scrutiny. This is crucial in full-range moves like high Kick with heel and Sweeping lotus leg. At striking speed, a flying limb (arm or leg), correctly actuated by the center, as distinct from by the limb itself, is inherently emptier than a slow-moving one.. The effort required to reproduce during several seconds, that which takes a tenth of that time, can obscure the finer intrinsic centered-ness of the limb. Why? Because a limb moving slowly away from the center requires more holding. (This in no way interferes with the practice-principle of releasing as much excess energy as possible) Thus sensing the core-line of an inactive limb can be learned, and then applied to a series of ever more energetic renditions of a particular move.

A lifetime of locomotion whose form ignores and even abuses the natural centered-ness of human limbs is a powerful habit that constantly and insidiously seeks to re-establish itself. Habits are very good at what they do. One of Cheng's devices (as I understand it) for sensing both the center-line and an empty leg is the peeling foot. This process manifests either from a back stance or a bow stance. The focus of attention is the rear foot as the body moves forward.

In the absence of a thrusting back leg or a rising body center, the rear knee tends to fall. It must not be lifted nor moved backward by unintended muscle action. As the process continues into the front foot, the rear knee hangs. That means the energy is downward not forward. It may move forward with the body-center, but you are not deliberately bringing the thigh forward. The corollary of this action is synchronous suspension of the leg from the hip-joint and peeling of the foot-sole from the ground.

The latter action likens the curved-not-folded sole to a self-stick postage stamp peeling from its backing.

In form practice, the leg will continue moving to its required destination. But by sensing that hanging thigh just at the moment the tip of the foot is neither on nor off the ground, so to speak, you can get very close to understanding a truly empty leg. A flying leg is also free of torso-weight, but the energy of the move is clearly greater or noisier than a still, hanging limb. I've dwelt on this issue simply because many long-term practicers seem not to have succeeded in this endeavor, that is, emptying the massive amount of tissue in each leg.

As the foot-peeling leg empties, it does so along its center-line, which is closer to the bones than to where you may sense the bulk to be. Therefore the energy exits down the thigh through the center of the knee (The knee is not the knee-cap, which is where many indicate their knee to be), then the shank, ankle, and finally along the foot's center-line to the front tip. At this juncture, the foot will have just cleared the ground. If like most people, you're used to moving through or using your feet along some other, more diagonal, line, then close scrutiny is required to preserve the center-line. (Toe-out, equally heel-in, locomotion is very common in highly civilized populations; not so common in others)

Although slanting use of feet may seem like a non-problem, the foot-style is actually a flag of leg-style. When energy enters or leaves a foot diagonally, it signifies a collapsed or stressed leg structure above. In fact, sensing this tendency in a partner's or opponent's legs can be decisive. If the leg is already misaligned, it takes very little to send it on its way to the detriment of the owner's position.

Stances or steps wherein legs are at different angles, are components of most Tai Chi movement. It can prove useful to consider these structures as variations of, or deviations from, the intrinsic parallel-leg structure in locomotion or horse-stance. If we assign a cardinal direction to a bow-stance front leg, then the rear leg will be set at some inter-cardinal angle, whose size varies from 45 degrees to almost 90 degrees. Bow stances are at their most economical, it seems, when weight is centered between both whole feet. This weighting prevails when the front shank is vertical. Moving further forward with both heels on the ground signals confusion or a cardinal error. The center begins to fall as the front shank or lower-leg passes through vertical. If you engage with a partner/opponent while using a nominal bow stance then allow the front shank to move forward past vertical, you will suffer defeat, or your partner/opponent is just not skilful enough. Yes there are ways of correcting this error while engaging, but if you are evenly matched or the other is more skilful, a need to correct is a disadvantage. As usual, work with weapons will drive home the cardinal principle of not losing advantage.

You can now practice sensing the centered-ness of the foot-soles, that is, the legs, by maneuvering back and fore with or without pelvic rotation. Solo practice encourages undistracted scrutiny. Eventually, as in all Tai Chi movement, testing with play, especially at high stakes, will enforce structural seamless-ness in application. Study the different feel in each leg when the body center is oriented more toward one of them. None-the-less, each foot sole should maintain its center-line without one iota of thrust. Turning, and especially cranking, the pelvic girdle can attack knee alignment, causing lateral waving and possibly trauma. Resist any tendency to hold knees in place; practice leaving them where they are, correctly aligned or centered, while engaging in movement initiated at the center. This may take some scrutiny and practice, but in truth you have no choice if you wish to employ useful Tai Chi Chuan.

It is difficult to maintain center-lines in bow-stances, because one leg is aligned with the body's cardinal forward axis, and the other with an inter-cardinal angle. I refer here to Cheng Man-ching stances. Other Yang-style bow-stances use rear-foot angles up to 90 degrees from front cardinal. Low stances, used often in training but seldom in combat, exacerbate the difficulty. In a bow-stance wherein the front thigh is horizontal or close to it, the shank above the rear foot can reach a low angle. The foot is flat on the ground while the shank may present 45 degrees to the ground. It is very easy to lose control, or to forcibly invade the equanimity of a foot's center-line. There is a matter of supple ankles. Merely sitting in a low bow-stance is good practice, of course, but the integrity of the structure needs to be tested in both solo and partnered moves. When I am under repeated attack in partner-practice while merely defending for training purposes, I often explain maintaining position as sensing both foot-soles flat on the ground. No more, no less. In other words, my obliging attacker, by attacking my torso, is trying to dislodge me from where I am not. And as long as one maintains viable Tai Chi structure, an integrated torso, one really is not doing very much of anything, so there is little for another to get any purchase on.

Compared with bow-steps or -stances, parallel-footed moves are fairly simple. These include Cloud hands lateral stepping and Monkey rearward stepping. In the Cheng short form (I mean no dishonor to Cheng's insistence that it was Yang's form), the former maneuver maintains a horse-stance throughout its lateral motion. The legs do not cross, but are brought toward the other leg or placed away from it along a single line of direction. While sitting in one leg one extends the empty one laterally to a distance of about two shoulder-widths. Both legs maintain the foot-soles' center-lines. After trying many thousands of these and observing thousands more attempts, I can forgive a skeptical, Oh yeah? Says who? This step is much easier said than done. Are you sure that there is no shading of weight toward the inside edge of the empty leg?

But it is a parallel-footed step and thus is simpler than one with different leg, that is, foot, angles. What we are really faced with here is standing centered in one leg while the other is being extended equally centered at some distance from the body's overall center. It is essential, I could say absolutely, to sit on a centered limb if that is the only one you're standing on. Otherwise the practice is merely teaching you to engage structures that don't work. Furthermore, whatever your current sense of self-awareness, any uneven relaxation represents at least two tense regions, each working against the other, trying to stop you from falling. In other words, you can't get out of the exterior while you're (usually unknowingly) using bulk muscle to hold yourself up. Therefore, a centered full or empty limb is one that is equally relaxed but not collapsed along its length: the energy moves along the core. The core is smoothest and greatest when the limb, or any component of the body, is equally relaxed along the energy's pathway.

Centered legs are therefore difficult to attain if the body-center is out of plumb. Tilting or swaying the pelvis is an important source of uneven leg energy. Gravity is an energy that affects everything we do. And just as we align ourselves with gravity in, say, Wu Ji standing, so an aligned leg unattached to the torso could well stand without one iota of adjustment by bulk muscle. The leg would be centered because habit or tension is not interfering: intrinsic structure prevails. This is the structure through which intrinsic or instinctual energy flows. That is probably why effortless movement is said to be a corollary of empty physique. Thinking or consciousness has little to do with actuating intrinsic energy (How did you do that? Do What?). After several decades of contemplating movement, I'm led to venture that the thinking mind **is** exterior or bulk muscle. This makes sense to me because the exterior thinking-mind is in the same realm as exterior muscle, while the instinctual wisdom-mind resides with the sinews: the interior.

None of this changes when a limb is off the ground. Arms are already off the ground, and they can readily be sensed as balanced. Just let them hang. Finding the center-line of an arm becomes familiar from Wu Ji standing (See The Foundation), in which emptiness and stillness are the guides. Or one could apply weight and energy along the length of an arm, as in holding a light weight. The limb may be relatively straight, which is easier to work with, or it may be flexed. In partner practice or combat, a Tai Chi arm must be completely relaxed until contact, and during the split-second of a strike. The arm in this case is merely a conduit for what I call a yang pulse.

One of those words is actually redundant because yang and pulse have the same meaning in terms of Tai Chi energy. Yang energy **is** pulsar; even a push (a term not needed in Tai Chi Chuan) is a pulse. Perhaps meditating on a typical Tai Chi strike sequence of four-per-second will bring this issue into focus. (Meditating does not mean thinking) Thus an arm or a leg merely needs to allow the bullet of a yang pulse to pass through the barrel of the limb without interference. When you fire a gun it doesn't help to manipulate the barrel after you've pulled the trigger.

Exactly the same principles apply when the limb is moving laterally, as in, say, a backhander and Sweeping lotus leg. These movements include a relatively large amount of rotational energy engendered by a spinning central axis. If the limb is short, that is, flexed, at the beginning of the move, it may lengthen with inflationary or peng energy flowing along its central axis. The same process occurs in a wind sock in a stiff breeze. Clearly, one can fold and unfold an elbow or knee without impetus from the torso (Chapter 3). But it **is** Tai Chi practice to ensure that as the limb lengthens, the unfolding or lateral energy is secondary to the lengthening energy. And at full length, at any speed, folding energy must be a minor component of the whole. Otherwise, one could attack one's own elbow or knee by forcing it into lock. A joint that is too loose can yield the same result as the limb is snapped open by centrifugal energy. Tai Chi strikes and many other moves are soft whips, and like a whip, cannot fully manifest length if folding energy interferes. The same applies to one of those party devices that uncurl as you blow into it. These devices neatly demonstrate inflation-energy lifting or acting on a tube (a limb) merely by passing through its center.

Unless clearly intended, it is pointless and distracting to lift a limb in Tai Chi practice. An arm may rise, but that is because its rising energy originates **along** its length. Furthermore, because the end of a limb is susceptible to even small amounts of deflection-energy or indeed any invasive energy across its structure, both form and function need to be no less seamless than in short-range Tai Chi moves. Sweeping lotus leg is a long-limb technique throughout application. In other words, the knee is not flexed between ground and target. The flying leg is a spoke in the protoplasmic, elastic wheel of the rotating center. It has the whip-spring quality of a short fishing rod. The leg may flex, but only because it becomes shorter as it passes under the torso. It compresses under the influence of its own weight and peng energy. Therefore it flexes, but the intent is to maintain its length.

This is a high-energy move in Tai Chi's range. So the limb had better be centered along its length as it flies. A small deviation near the origin can deliver a big problem at maximum distance. The flying limb will arrive at cardinal, 45 degrees **maximum** from its initial orientation, a moment before the reflexing center begins its return journey. And at maximum energy, the limb will move from virtually vertical to more-or-less horizontal, while maintaining its soft, long form. If the leg moves above horizontal, it is because it's being lifted; the intent is hazy. You would have to lift the leg with itself , a no-no in principle, or move the center up or down during the movement. If that is intended, fine, but clarity is essential. So through the whole move, one is in effect swinging a slightly curved tube. A centered foundation, connection, and limb is essential during trial-and-error practice of such large moves. There is so much energy in play, that small errors become large misses because they are obscured by high noise-to-signal ratios.

Also, maintaining a horizontal leg in slow form is very physical, a dread word to internal artists. That is always the challenge and genius of slow practice: you have maximum opportunity the release excess energy. None-the-less, relatively fast, very loose, practice has its lessons about overall feel and inner form, including the limb's center-line. This centered-ness will, of course, remain a mystery unless one intends to first find it and then keep it. Low-energy practice, such as when the leg flies only a quarter of its range, is not only beneficial, but is closer to the parameters of most applications at speed.

Finally, the centered-ness of the standing limb, any move's foundation, had better be maintained, had it not? Lateral attack of the knee by excess energy from neglect or trying too hard, is not what a knee is made to withstand. Obvious to the intellect, this principal seems to be most students' major distraction in swinging-limb practice. Therefore do not twist the knee. Any amount is too much. In general, which is as near to always as you get in Tai Chi practice, don't allow energy to move into or out of a knee other than along its pure cardinal center-line.

3

HINGING AND ROTATION
Distinguished partners
Shaping the frame for action

How does the human body move? Well, according to how it's made in terms of frame and joints. Muscles are there to serve the bones: that's a guiding principle in realizing what your body is doing when you move it, when "it" moves. When bodies lose weight they're eventually left with skin and bone, so to speak. In other words, muscle goes a lot faster than the rest. Also, under conditions of sustained economy, muscle that was once bulky reduces to virtual sinew, the material of tendons and ligaments. So in motion and manipulation, how the bones move relative to each other forms the core for shaping the body in action. The art of manipulating others' bodies (not the main subject here) is based on this simple principle.

As with universal core principles, yin-ness and yang-ness, all of human movement comprises the quintessential components of hinging and rotation. We have two large sets of hinges, knees and elbows, which don't really favor any other kind of action. These joints are to all intents and purposes pure hinges: they have a single direction. Hand and foot digits are hinges, and it feels that ribs, at least in parts, also hinge. Otherwise, all other joints are universal, like hips and shoulders, or are mixed, like spine, ankles, wrists, palms and foot-arches, and less visible structures, such as clavicle, ribs, pelvis, and scapulas.

As hinges, knees, elbows, and digits are simple in principle: they move like a **pinned** door-hinge. But in principle does not mean in practice; civilization and undemanding lifestyles have seen to that. It becomes obvious from even cursory observation of human movement that hinged joints are not used as such. This is especially true in legs, which carry body-weight through a huge number of steps in a lifetime. Knees (and elbows) are commonly over-flexed to the point of locking, allowing force to be lodged in them. Knees are commonly misaligned with the direction in which a body intends to proceed. Toe-out foot alignment due to collapsed hip-joints, and its apparent twin, heel-in contraction, is so common in civilized people (Chapter 2) that those with natural, functional alignment may be treated with correctional footwear.

Thus a would-be Tai Chi practicer may bear a complex array of habits. These present progress as a matter of not doing things to which they have grown accustomed. Perhaps that's one of the meanings of the adage: A thousand start, but one finishes. Yet not doing Tai Chi is so much more difficult than doing it. And that is why I warn students that they have two bodies, one habitual and one natural. Engaging the core components of natural movement is one way of finding a simple, though not easy, solution to this entanglement.

Examining body structure and movement is useless without setting a foundation for estimation and scrutiny. In this case that foundation is in centered legs and proper Tai Chi conditions at the body center. Feet sit flat on the ground, the weight sensed evenly front-to-back and side-to-side. This weighting can vary front-to-back, mostly in two-footed structures like the bow-stance. Side-to-side is, in this book, immutably even, especially when only part of a foot is weighted, as in back- and front-stances. Sensing balance in the foot-soles is applied at all levels of practice. But it is important to remember that feet are just the ends of legs. Using them like flags to sense energy is very useful only if it becomes internalized by repetition of the right signals. You'll know about this when you no longer have to check for centered-ness; instead you'll tend to switch to noting error beginning to edge in. The object, other than having a good time, is to cultivate competence, not to pursue perfection.

Hinging and rotation each has two basic means of actuation. One is movement seated in the limb itself, such as using biceps et al to hinge an arm, or rotating a leg on the toe-pad while the torso is still. The other basic method is using a moving body to flex or rotate a limb joint or member while the limb-part is still. This method occurs as follows: Touch some still object or surface with fingertips of an extended arm. Leave the fore-arm where it is, and flex the elbow by moving the torso toward the hand. The suggestion to flex an elbow without moving the fore-arm, has foxed a lot of people, even experienced martial artists, though they may have used the technique many times.

Rotating a leg with the body is very common in Tai Chi stepping (and in a daughter art, Bagua, in which the round-seeking principle dominates). Merely rotating the center while in a back stance with the front heel-pad on the ground will re-orient that front leg to the center's new direction. It's done: the leg has rotated without itself doing anything except maintain its original connection to the torso. Pretty much all Tai Chi movement thus comprises mixtures of hinging and rotation, each varied by interplay of limbs and torso, periphery and center.

It doesn't seem to be common in Western cultures to consider the largest hinge in the human body: what in Chinese sounds like kwa. It is the hinge between thighs and torso. The crease between abdomen and thigh (one or both) is an external flag for this huge joint. Sinking a vertical torso into flexing legs steadily increases this hinge and its external fold. Also, raising a leg, empty from the knee down, as in Golden rooster, is another actuation of this joint.

A core concern in Tai Chi motion is, how much are joints used ? Economy, which I construe as Tai Chi's most basic principle, would suggest first: as little as possible, while doing what is necessary. Since most people use arms more than legs, let's consider elbows first. When an elbow flexes the arm shortens. De-flexing an elbow increases the angle between upper- and lower-arm, thus lengthening or opening the arm. When de-flexed to excess an elbow locks; when fully flexed the fore-arm lies as if collapsed adjacent to the upper part. Experience answers the question, How much? with answers to two others: In what form are arms most viable? And intrinsically strongest?

My answer is the same for each of these: in its middle range of flexure, as in the posture Raise hands or its look-alike, Play the pipa. Here, the back elbow is close to a right angle (90 degrees), and the forward one at about 120 degrees. Both upper-arms are angled forward, as in all active Tai Chi structures. Elbows moving back behind the torso's lateral line, which runs vertically between shoulder and hip joints, is a low-priority move. Each elbow flexure is viable in both directions. One may fold a little more without rendering the elbow more closed than open. The other may open more or de-flex until the arm reaches its maximum functional length, as in the pendent arms of Ready. In this latter form arms are curved, and may yet lengthen a little by resting them empty on the thighs' lateral lines, as in Wu Ji (The Foundation).

Thus arms are viable between elbow flexures of about 90 degrees and 165 degrees (although joint-flexure is not in practice a matter of measuring angles). They are at their most viable in the middle range, perhaps the middle two-thirds or three-quarters. They are at their useful limit at each end of this range. At the short limit, a lower-arm is rendered redundant, and the elbow-joint becomes the functional end of the arm, as in Elbow-stroke or Folding. In the long arm, it is strongest along its length, as in Piercing (empty-hand or weapons, such as sword). The long arm can also be applied radially, that is, across its length, but elbow flexure is not a significant component of the action. The curve of the whole arm is maintained until contact.

Problems arise during upper-limb movements when hinging and rotation are not clearly distinguished. It's important that intent and deed are aligned along the whole arm. When the intention or requirement is for a fore-arm to rotate, it is important that the result does no unknowingly lift an elbow or collapse a shoulder-joint. The former occurs when the effort to rotate exceeds the fore-arm's ability to do so. This excess energy then actuates the upper-arm away from the torso, lifting the elbow in the process. In the other case, wherein the palm rotates upward (as in patting something upward), the intent to rotate should not exceed the fore-arms' ability. Here the upper-arm is forced toward the torso; or the shoulder-joint collapses, as if holding something under the arm. This is ok for newspapers, bad for Tai Chi practice.

Similarly, the intention to hinge a wrist aligning the hand's center digit with the fore-arm can instead yield a wrist also hinged laterally (one of its properties as a semi-universal joint). This is because a habit of applying excess energy to movements has over-powered one's ability to sense what's really happening. In other words, rotate the forearm softly, meanwhile ensuring that the elbow maintains its position; do not hold the elbow in place, just leave it there. There is a fundamental difference between holding a position and maintaining it: one tends to be external, the other internal. This movement or hand-form is prevalent in suspended arms especially when the fore-arm has rotated the palm upward, as in Holding-the-ball or Embrace tiger. The palm is not rotating itself: it is an action of the fore-arm. Persuading students that a hand is merely the end of an arm can be difficult in a culture where hands are deemed to be doing so much.

If elbows get twisted out of alignment because of excess fore-arm rotation, at least the elbows don't suffer trauma, unless another person is administering the arm-rotation. Knees are another matter entirely. Twisted knees and knees levered laterally across their natural alignment seem common in general life and in Tai Chi practice. This observation includes Tai Chi literature, in pictures of teachers and masters demonstrating postures such as Snake creeps down. This form is often chosen for demonstration because it is a difficult structure close to the edge of Tai Chi practice. All the more reason to ensure that one is not attacking oneself with excess effort nor by excess teaching.

Basically, Snake creeps down or Squatting whip is a back-stance. And in a back-stance the weighted leg, in which you're standing or sitting, is at some angle from the body's external cardinal nose-and-navel direction. This angle is in general a maximum of 45 degrees. Cheng Man-ching's requirement in form practice is sometimes to point the leg in one cardinal direction, and to rotate the body-center toward the next cardinal, 90 degrees away. That's training. If you need to move deep down into the back leg of a bow-stance, then it's best to rotate the leg outward (on its heel) to the cardinal from its more usual corner or inter-cardinal. This time the angle is a very practical matter. Try dropping deep into the back leg maintaining a vertical torso: you will only get so far down before knee hinge and ankle hinge reach their reasonably viable limit.

Now try the same move after first rotating the 45-degree leg to 90 degrees from the torso's original direction. You won't have to go down over a too-hinged knee or a heavily compressed ankle. The body/torso should be allowed to "follow" the leg; it will rotate about 45 degrees toward the leg's direction. In other words, you're letting yourself down laterally, with the torso placed inside the back leg, as distinct from over the leg's center. In all the moves here described (and throughout my Tai Chi practice) the center-lines of the limbs, easily sensed in the foot-soles, are maintained. Period. Exactly, precisely, without the slightest deviation.

Otherwise two problems will arise: twisting, lateral levering, or both, in the knee. Twisting occurs usually because the torso is rotated to excess away from its natural alignment with a leg or legs. In other words, the shank of the weighted leg is subjected to rotation that should stop within the thigh. Turning the torso in either direction should have no effect on knees; the knees stay aligned with the feet. What happens when torso-turning is overdone is that this twisting energy forces knees outward or inward; there is no longer a smooth alignment of hip, knee, and ankle/foot. Everyday locomotion using (actually abusing) legs at an angle from the body's cardinal direction obscures this sense of misalignment, and muffles the feeling of knees being used other than in the body's intended direction. Who even notices anything wrong in placing a foot on the ground with a straight, almost locked, knee; making initial ground contact with the rear edge of the foot, so that the foot points up and outward; then moving through the foot diagonally from the back corner-edge to the front large toe-ball, mashing the joint in the process?

The modern human body still does its best to compensate for this ill-use, and people seem able to move about to their satisfaction. There is little demand on natural human structure and abilities from the smooth, even surfaces of civilization. Also, self-abuse is encouraged by footwear that has little to do with natural and healthy human feet. Imagine the general response to being offered gloves which jam the fingers into a tight cone. Unfortunately, such practical matters are rendered redundant at an early age by adult fashion and its attack on natural structure. By the time someone is considering Tai Chi practice there are decades of bad habits in place and internalized.

So in Squatting whip, an edge-of-the-body maneuver, extreme damage to knees is possible if any of those old habits remain. Hence the emphasis in Tai Chi practice is always on relaxation, but within Tai Chi structure. To relax out of Tai Chi structure is to collapse. To force your way out of structure is, well, the use of force. It matters not who administers that force, it still violates Tai Chi principle. Conserving structure is a matter of first finding it. This is an internal understanding but can be taught or acquired or merely recognized by a body realizing itself.

To maintain Tai Chi or intrinsic structure, one first needs to sense it. Then you'll know what it is you mean to conserve. This is no flippant aphorism; the energy of conserving is for most students conflated with the energy of trying. The former is more instinctual, more internal; the latter is usually a conscious muscular process. I would go further: even thinking of doing something will activate exterior muscles. Who concerns themselves with maintaining an upright structure in everyday life, as I do while standing at this computer keyboard? It is, even for civilized humans, an internalized process. But the body is not still. It is constantly adjusting for deviation even in still exercises, such as Wu Ji.

If your attention is first in the alignment of a centered knee or elbow, then relaxed movement maintaining this alignment is, in essence, internal practice. Also, letting an elbow remain still in a relaxed arm while the fore-arm is being rotated, characterizes internal practice. These are processes of some delicacy for beginners. They are also typical in an experienced Tai Chi practicer, and reflect an essential difference between doing and maintaining.

It is essential to sense as gross distortion of Tai Chi structure, knees forced out of alignment, and elbows pushed against the torso, a move which also closes off the upper-arm-torso connection. One begins by first sensing their relaxed starting positions. In fact, sensing a soft touch of fingers-tips on a wall or still (later, moving) partner, while moving back and fore is really quite simple, although the process of that maintenance is quite complex.

Finally in this context, there's the forceful collapse of knees because of squatting. This is distinct from flexing the whole leg. There seems to be confusion among practicers about the difference between an inactive structure and an active, Tai Chi, one. In Snake creeps down or Squatting whip it is tempting, perhaps because of an ability to let go in general, to drop the hip joint below the knee. In this case the thigh will slope down toward the torso, primarily erect in a viable structure. Legs are distinct from and similar to arms. Also, they are out of sight and larger, thus occupying some more obscure realm. When studying legs it is often favorable to first look at arms. They are mostly weightless and anyway much more within our attention.

An arm tends to stop rising when the upper-arm reaches horizontal; a Tai Chi elbow is reluctant to rise, and very reluctant to rise above a shoulder. What, after all, is up there? Put before you the other body, combatant or partner, and test how far a practical move can take the elbow upwards. Bear in mind that principles of general practice apply here. Of course one can go beyond this guideline as the situation demands. But fluid flow between torso and arm is fundamentally different when that fluid, energy and substance, gravitates toward the body. Also, the energy supporting the arm switches from being mainly tensile to partially compressive. This is because the arm is leaning or resting on the shoulder when that arm is above it. And that is why it feels so different to maintain an arm rising vertically from the shoulder, compared with an arm hanging from it. Each offers its own challenges in relaxation. But the internal energy pattern is quite distinct in each. Even a Western physiologist would record different patterns of energy distribution in comparative thermographs, a method for measuring activity by recording heat.

There is good reason to bring a suspended arm up to shoulder-height, as in the Opening move of several internal arts forms. From fully pendent up to horizontal uses one type of energy, gravity. This extends the limb along its length, then hangs on the limb as it moves higher up toward horizontal. Beyond that, gravity is felt as mass down through the arm toward the shoulder. This is a matter of practical sensing, not physics theory.

Raising a vertical, active arm up to horizontal has a structural counterpart in a standing leg, as it moves from being essentially vertical, to the thigh becoming horizontal as the body is lowered. The torso remains vertical during Squatting whip or similar moves. There is no need to cant or lean the torso, though many do this, usually unwittingly. The thigh engages the same general pattern of energy-use as it moves down from a slightly flexed angle to horizontal. When the hip joint falls below the knee, the leg as a whole engages a pattern of inaction or collapse. The bulk of the rear thigh is now resting or leaning on the bulk of the rear calf.

Rising from this position involves a different set of springs from those used to rise when a hip is above the knee.

Again, this is not a matter of theory; since there is none in Tai Chi practice. Explanations of what is actually happening or what is sensed internally is another matter. The viability of any Tai Chi process or structure is very easily tested by others. An opponent or partner, more importantly the former, can prevail over a squatting person with a single finger. That is hardly the case with a person sitting in a leg compressed to horizontal thigh. The difference between the active potential of the two structures is like that between yes and no. Generally, leg-use moves through the middle range of flexure, as in other Tai Chi maneuvers. But realizing the limits is just as important as knowing the middle ground. How can one stay within limits and away from the edges otherwise? According to the Classics, all moves shall be comfortable.

Almost all Tai Chi moves are combinations of simple flexing, one aspect of the straight, and rotation, one view of the round. Two hinges may be engaged simultaneously; the same for two rotations. In all moves these combinations unfold or develop synchronously. In other words, a hinge will open or close to the same degree as that of a rotation. If an elbow moves through 10 degrees and the fore-arm pivots through 20 degrees in a move, then the latter will have rotated 10 degrees when the former has hinged five degrees, and so on. In this case, one degree of elbow, two degrees of fore-arm.

The relationship is not always linear as in this example. The degree of change in each component is more usually linked by a curved or spiral relationship, but that's too complex to explain succinctly in my words. The classical adage, All parts arrive at once, sets out the relationships at start and finish. What happens in between has more to do with the 10,000 variations of Yin and Yang, or here in the quintessential components of movement, hinging and rotation.

Such accounts as this one neatly illustrate a reverse aphorism I use, which is that Tai Chi is easier done than said. Nonetheless, I'll try to address the tricky subject of how energy changes in an arm (or flying leg) as it gets longer. What I am saying is that longitudinal energy needs to prevail more and more as a limb gets longer.

One view of an arm getting longer is an increasing elbow-joint angle. Another view is the increasing distance between finger-tips and shoulder. It soon becomes obvious to the thinking-mind, that the angle and distance refer to the same tendency: one increases as does the other. Confusion arises in the application of energy to achieve this movement. Lengthening an arm comprises both penetrating energy in the finger-tips and slapping energy in the back-hand.

Let's look first at penetrating energy. When an elbow is maximally folded, say at about 90 degrees, back-hand energy is more important as the joint opens or unfolds. Similarly, palm energy manifests as the arm is again folded. If penetrating or stabbing energy is needed when the arm is folded, then we can use the shoulder-joint and torso rotation to propel the fore-arm along its length. If one adopts the form of holding, say, a soccer ball with vertical palms just in front of the torso, pivoting the center or pelvic girdle first one way then the other will drive each fore-arm forward, delivering piercing energy through the finger-tips.

In other words, as the right hip moves forward the right arm will do the same. The left arm and hip move back at the same time. That illustrates the stabbing aspect of the movement. This type of action can be extended simply by letting the elbow-joint open until the arm is obviously pointing away from the torso. If you now return to the original ball-holding position, you can again rotate the pelvis, but this time ensuring that elbows maintain their distance from the torso. Now you would be merely swinging the ball from side to side. Here, the energy is lateral, as in clapping the hands.

You may now extend an arm by pointing with the finger tips. Starting with the original structure, but without the ball, the fore-arm will move, from about 45 degrees to both forward and lateral body cardinals, to being straight in front of that arm's shoulder. In the same move, the back-hand will have swung outward. That is, you could penetrate with the finger-tips and slap outwards with the back-hand using the same movement. Easier done than said.

The purpose of this is to observe that in any moment slapping with the back-hand is a different intent from piercing with the finger-tips. And it is very important that the intent to unhinge the elbow-joint doesn't lock it, or even get near, during engagement with partner or opponent. Therefore, when an arm is long, as it is when it's hanging, lateral energy should not force the elbow-joint to attack itself. This seems very obvious in words or as a concept, but is a common confusion in practice.

If, therefore, you apply unhinging energy to an elbow when the arm is long, you risk damage to the joint. This is especially important when the long arm is downward, because 1: the elbow can get too straight, 2: the elbow can be forced toward the torso, thus closing off the shoulder-joint, 3: the palm is often rotated forward-and-up as the back-hand is slapped down to deflect or attack an approaching body part. (The arm can then re-hinge in a reflex to address the space in front of the body center, as is often needed in competitive or combative close engagement) It is also important not to push with shoulder-movement or use the shoulder at all to extend an unfolding arm. A shoulder, as part of the torso, may initiate the move, but it does that only once as part of a yang pulse.

So as the arm gets longer, the energy along it becomes increasingly important. At the limit the energy is mostly longitudinal. That way, the unfolding energy of the arm, useful as it is in the mid-range, does not lead to elbow damage or error in tactics. To all intents and purposes, unfolding or unhinging energy is redundant in a straight arm. Bear in mind that extending a whole arm combines both piercing and unhinging energies. The problems arise when the practicer is not clear in applying these complementary counter-parts. For example, many Tai Chi moves simultaneously harness the lateral energy of an arm to deflect, as the front end of the arm, say the fingers, attacks with piercing energy. It is precisely these kinds of combination that render a Tai Chi fighter both difficult to get at and to get away from. But the components need to be seamlessly balanced and always complementary.

Although legs have structures closely similar to those of arms, they seem to be treated quite differently from them by moving bodies. There is a notable difference because legs bear body-weight while arms are pendent from the torso. Locomotion infant-style is quadrupedal, but in adults is more legs-helped-by-arms, a sort of two-plus-two relationship. But when it comes to moving limbs through space, the differences are reduced simply because these movements employ intrinsic structure. Thus a hip pivots like a shoulder, a knee hinges like an elbow, an ankle moves like a wrist, and feet manipulate like hands, though less so.

An important difference lies in the ability of a fore-arm to rotate. Whereas a fore-arm can rotate a hand as much as 180 degrees, the lower leg has no such ability: knee and foot point in the same direction. Therefore all foot-turning is seated in a hip-joint, in torso-turning, or in both.

Legs and arms in Tai Chi motion, whether locomoting or manipulating, begin movement at the torso. Energy then moves through elbow and wrist or knee and ankle. The simplest example of this in legs is Flying lotus leg and its analogs. Here, the main energy is across the substance of the leg as it arcs upward from the ground to horizontal maximum (See previous notes on arm orientation). In other words, the foot at the end of such a leg usually delivers the foot's outer side. The tip and the foot-sole are redundant. This is analogous with an arm-move delivering the small-finger edge of the hand. There is a difference. A horizontal hand-edge has an elbow joint behind it oriented about 45 degrees from the vertical. An arm palm-up in front of the shoulder has a vertically-aligned elbow behind it: the point of the elbow faces downward. When a leg is flying radially, the knee-cap is uppermost, its hinge horizontal; the knee is oriented to the vertical. When contact is made, therefore, the lateral energy of the move applies across the knee-joint. This, also, can be damaging to the joint because of ligament and tendon trauma. But it is different from trauma sustained by locking the hinge.

Another structural error that can invade the move's effectiveness is unwittingly rotating the leg so that the toes turn outward. Letting the heel lead slightly is not a problem, so long as that is the intent. My understanding of an effective Lotus leg is that the leg begins long, behind the torso, and resting through its length on the whole toe-pad. The front leg is oriented 45 degrees maximum from the intended target, and the foot of this leg forms a letter-T bar to the leg suspended behind it. As the torso rotates toward the target from its initial 45 degrees maximum, the back leg is swept passed it and toward the target. The flying leg remains long. In other words, don't hinge the knee or kwa. If the energy is clean enough it will project the foot as high as the hip, maximum. This is a good example of hip joints' universal property.

This is not necessarily a kick: trying to kick is a distraction from the move's versatility. Any part of the leg along its length may engage with the other body. Trauma is avoided by striking the surface of the target, rather than attempting something more forceful. The latter practice is sure to lead to either damage or upset: yours. The other main leg move, Kick with heel, begins when the leg is already up with the knee opposite the hip, as in Golden rooster. This height is also a maximum: the move has many uses much closer to the ground. The flick-like pulse of the torso-center toward the target sends the foot away from the hip with longitudinal energy. The target is struck by the foot sole, especially the heel. It is important not to distract this energy with thrusting, which pushes the knee backward. The effectiveness of this move, as in all Tai Chi strikes, is in the range and appropriately brief energy-pulse. So, again, the hinge is opening because of energy, a pulse of energy, moving through the limb along its length. It's quite simple in principle and in practice if one generates a single pulse;

its elastic reflex inheres in the original intent. And the corollary to this is do one thing at a time, time passing at tenths of a second. This time-scale helps explain why Tai Chi Chuan in invisible to an external observer. At any speed movements need the clarity inherent in seamless melding of hinging and rotation.

Finally on this subject, I suggest that one universal joint should not be used at all. This is the delicate joint between head and neck. Let it float, then maintain its alignment throughout practice. Don't try to lengthen it, as in Hold the head erect, or Look straight ahead. Hold nothing: merely maintain its slight curve at the top of the spine. And don't look straight ahead with the vision parallel to the ground. Where, after all, is your opponent, or your future? Close to the ground. Cheng Man-ching suggested that the nose and navel stay in line, and that seems to be sufficient. Aligning the head-joint relates to a body vertically below. Beware the horizon.

4

TO RAISE THE TOE...

...Is to raise the heel
Joined in the sole

A human's basic relationship with the Earth is founded where the soles of feet meet the ground. This statement of the obvious would be redundant were it not that modern humans are programmed from a young age to ignore it. Tai Chi practice persuades us that it can be very difficult to recapture this Common Sense. Inherited body structures and patterns of use plus modern life-style, especially footwear and sitting, insulate and detach us from the very ground we seem designed to stand on and move over. Although a competent Tai Chi body can manifest a certain amount of inflationary (peng) energy, and even condensing and adhering energies, while that body is airborne, its full compendium of resources is severely limited. Human feet are attracted to the ground, and have evolved to feel their way across it.

And so to another obvious statement: a foot has its best relationship with the ground when it's on it. In any demanding situation, such as in primitive conditions, a foot that joins with the ground needs all of its intrinsic attributes to cope. A body's balance and viability depend on this foundation (Chapter 2 addresses some of this). A foot-sole has two basic components, and these parts need to maintain a relationship throughout locomotion, and especially while the body is under test or attack. An intrinsic component of a foot's basic relationship with the ground is the close relationship between the rear and front active centers of the foot-sole. I call these centers the heel-pad and toe-pad. They are pads, not balls.

In other words, they are flat cushions, each of which, when fully engaged, can readily support the body's weight and engage in diverse maneuvers. However, each pad and both pads work best when the foot-sole is in one piece. The foot-sole is more flat than curved. The more curved it is, the more angular it becomes, especially in flexure. At the limit, the front pad is folded in half: the structure when the rest of the sole is about vertical and the digits sit in the ground. In the more general mid-range, the angle between heel-pad and toe-pad is quite large; that is, the sole is relatively flat. Modern practices of using the rear edge of the foot, and thrusting while walking, can present steep angles between foot and ground.

The former practice has a lot to do with striding in hard footwear. Thus the rear edge of the forward foot comes crashing to the ground insulated by hard shoes or cushions, which seem designed to encourage this type of locomotion. Over a lifetime of this, ankles, knees, which are often locked, and lower back can sustain many thousands of shocks for which they are not designed. But that's another story. Thrusting comes readily in a pushy world where being in a hurry is viewed as an attribute. Both habits force feet to present steep angles to the ground, whether approaching it or leaving it.

Tai Chi practice and demanding environments require competence before style. In fact natural movement is much less idiosyncratic than modern habits. In other words, humans could be much less distinguishable by gait than they are. Thus learning to move according to Tai Chi principles reduces the differences between humans without in any way interfering with personal versatility and talent. When one is engaging such human attributes, the action demands competence. And what one soon learns is the need for moving along the ground. Horizontally. With an erect torso. This is virtually impossible when one is thrusting up or falling down, for that is what many are doing when walking. Any half-competent Tai Chi student will topple effortlessly a body moving this way.

The solution to this and other problems is to relax legs so that the foot soles engage softly with the ground or body or weapon, and adhere to that surface between steps. This type of foot also tends to maintain a relatively flat sole. These parameters relate to horizontal movement, not undulating movement. If you move down or up during Tai Chi engagement your partner or opponent is going to ensure that your seeming wish is fulfilled. Yes, Tai Chi moves include intended lowering and elevating the body; as long as you know what you're doing, it's not a problem. What is important is that all moves are guided by strategy, not useless habit. And the horizontal, so to speak, is a corollary of that strategy.

When we consider the foot-sole in this context it becomes obvious that each pad is most useful when it is more or less flat, not more or less round: hence pad not ball. A long, slow spin on either pad will demonstrate this. Note that a fast spin can be made on almost any part of a foot, but may not be viable in action. Tai Chi spins are not necessarily slow, but they are stable and seamlessly interchangeable with other moves. Steps forward and back at various angles are the bread and butter of Tai Chi movement, the primary choice being forward.

In this case, a body-weighted leg is the foundation of the move; empty leg means empty of torso weight, not its own weight, which is considerable. Therefore the empty foot-sole seeks the ground inquisitively; it must in effect be asking a question. Is there anything here, for example? Or, What is the nature of the surface? Practicing on elevated structures, such as bricks and poles, in the dark (Care!), soon conveys the sense of these questions. In practice, and after plenty of it, this sensing is timeless and versatile, allowing seamless and decisive stepping at any speed. Thinking is too slow and too late. Forward stepping therefore presents a soft sole almost parallel with the ground. And because there is no reaching in Tai Chi practice (Cheng Man-ching: Don't be greedy), that step will be a modest one. Short steps are fast steps rapidly changing to suit the situation. Equilibrium is readily invaded when a leading foot moves forward with a large angle between sole and ground. Or simply because the foot is lifted prior to being put down. What is the point of this indecisive stepping?

When a foot goes down well, the heel-pad is flat on the ground. This sensible and viable approach can be interrupted by pulling back the digits, or any shortening of the top of a foot. Thus the toe-pad is also seeking the ground, and in a relaxed forward foot is never more than about a half-inch from it. This proximity does not preclude a foot or part of it engaging with another's lower limb: it just depends what the moment requires. A front foot can also apply the whole sole. And the toe-pad is often actuated in moves such as White crane and foot sweeps. Again, the sole tends to hug the horizontal, though is these cases, it will be traveling toward your body-center or in a short arc close to it.

Backward stepping is not Tai Chi practice's first choice. If one of two equally-matched opponents is moving back, he or she is at a strategic disadvantage. But Tai Chi Chuan being what it is, practicers train to move backward in the best way possible. As with forward moving, knees are flexed enough to allow a relaxed foot onto the ground; the heel is not lifted, toes are not pulled back, knees are not hardened, and the limb is centered (Chapter 2). For training, allow the whole of the retreating foot-sole onto the ground before shifting weight. This applies to an angled leg or one parallel to the standing leg. However, weight enters the foot toe-pad first, until the foot is centered front-to-back. This is the placement usually described as centered on the Bubbling Well, an acupuncture orifice a.k.a. Kidney 1. Clearly there are many shades of weighting in general practice. But equally, there are three main ones: whole foot, heel-pad, and toe-pad.

In Tai Chi back-stepping, therefore, a foot touches the ground toe-pad first, not digits first. The foot is suspended over the ground or surface so that the whole pad can easily engage. This move applies equally to angled and straight stepping. Then the weight moves along the center-line into the whole foot, regardless of angle. In some applications rearward stepping may move only as far as the toe-pad. This allows the body or leg to either rotate on the pad, or to open or de-flex. The former option allows the body to spin or the leg to rotate to some desired or required angle. The second case allows the body to reflex forward without engaging the whole foot-sole. A leg's braided spring-like structure extends through the foot-arch to the toe-pad, in other words, the far active center of a foot-sole, which in turn is the end of a leg. The heel-pad is the near active center of a foot-sole, and expresses energy more characteristic of the leg's core.

Backward locomotion requires legs parallel with the body's main direction. (The principle of this alignment is applied even in backward stepping round a circle. The intent is to place the new foot parallel with the main direction. This circle can be small in close maneuvers) Modern bodies seem to have difficulty with this parallel alignment. Toes appearing to point outward also means heels forced or contracted inward. So you'll need to maintain an open lower back by pointing straight back with the rear edge or prow of the heel. It may feel strange at first, but so what? Cheng's pithy observation was that if you step back for Repulse monkey with toes pointing out, then you have no idea what you are doing. That was good enough for me.

There is a third type of stepping, which actually overlaps with fore and back: cross-stepping. Basically, cross-stepping is an extension of Cloud-hands stepping, in which parallel feet move to either side but don't cross each other. It's a type of shuffle or half step. Cheng Man-ching's form (which he insisted was Yang's) exhibits no overt cross-stepping, though it is implied in diagonal forward steps as in Deflect. Here, the front-stepping foot pivots outwards on the heel-pad, such that it has a diagonal alignment with the rear-foot toe-pad, as distinct from heel-pad. In other words, the new foot moves somewhat laterally across the line of the standing or back foot.

Side-stepping itself brings a leg across the front or back of the standing leg, causing the body to move more or less along the shoulder-line. It is important as a foundational practice not to cross the legs such that the crotch becomes angular, rather than rounded. Cross-stepping is not viable without well-flexed knees. The aim is to present the whole foot-sole to the ground; the steps are thus inherently modest. To reach is an error in principle. Reaching allows only the edge of a foot to engage the ground. Also, entering a new foot diagonally through the corner of its heel in front-stepping, or diagonal front-corner (across the small digits) in rear-stepping, signals an unstable leg, a ropey foundation. In rapid lateral stepping, wherein front and back cross-stepping alternate, the toe-pad only may engage the ground. This is viable so long as the center-lines of the feet are maintained (Chapter 2). In general, it's good training to cross-step into the whole sole, noting that the new foot may be aligned with the torso's original orientation, or with some new angle (toe out or toe in, by rotating the leg via the heel-pad). Bagua, Tai Chi Chuan's daughter art, emphasizes this type of stepping, whereas Tai Chi Chuan applies such steps as part of its general repertoire.

Partner-practice and especially higher-stakes engagements can demonstrate and prove the viability of the foot-soles' close relationship with the ground. In essence, such practice is merely realizing a foot's real role, which is as the end of a leg. Jacking up heels and lifting the leg with the top of the foot are clearly the periphery dictating to the center. Tai Chi Chuan's principles are equally clearly at odds with such practices. Finally, I am not suggesting that the edges or rims of the feet can not be used in Tai Chi Chuan; one does what is necessary. But that, at least for now, is another story.

5

SIMILAR LIMBS
Modesty is the best policy
How not to get bent out of shape

What does an integrated body feel like? Or, How should my body feel? These and similar questions come my way often enough to put me on my toes, so to speak. My answer to both is a fudge because the truth isn't very helpful: I have no idea. Better answers to both questions are explorations, in other words, more questions.

A word picture of my own body these days is a tough, I hope not thick, elastic outer membrane encasing an oily, mobile-yet-elastic, homogeneous fluid. I don't feel joints as such. Nor do I sense anything between one part of my body and another. If my arm happens to be touching someone, and she or he moves, the inner touchline seems to connect directly to my foot-soles. The direction of the impinging energy is not an issue. So my self-portrait also turns out to be not very helpful: a me-shaped balloon.

Furthermore, my feet seem to ooze unglamorously along the ground; hardly an image of the fearsome martial artist. Nonetheless, maintenance of this rather bizarre inner state has helped me coax my body toward seamless Tai Chi movement.

Let's consider a state of integration, as distinct from its process. If you are integrated, what follows is redundant. Otherwise, the most integrated state is when you are still except to conserve the vital interior. Wu Ji standing is the nearest activity to this state, and that is why it is what it is (The Foundation). Any external move renders a more diffuse structure.

From directly overhead, a Wu Ji body looks like an oval, a little more wide than long. There are, of course, many body-types and -shapes, but an oval more or less summarizes the variations. Outward movement will add a pod to this oval: it is, after all, a budding move, as in an amoeba. It doesn't matter what is moving, arm or leg or both. One or more buds will extend the periphery of the oval in the intended direction. If the image is in outline, a rising upper arm or leg will appear as a growing pod until either reaches horizontal. Then the pod will begin to diminish as the end of the limb moves closer to the torso. If the move is continued, the arm pod will eventually disappear. The leg, even with the thigh adjacent to the upper torso, will present a protuberance.

The main issue is that Tai Chi moves tend to send energy **along** a limb, a process shown by the expanding pod. Many observers do not see this, however. What they often think they see is someone **lifting** an arm or leg or whatever. Well, the limb can **rise** devoid of any intent to lift it. If the limb were a wind-sock, a breeze passing through it would fill it with inflationary (peng) energy, causing the limb to become horizontal as the breeze strengthened. This is a simple and common example of how energy moving through a limb may cause it to rise. If the wind-sock is sagging or folded, the breeze's flow also will inflate it to more or less cylindrical.

A Tai Chi-body is similarly inflated, but with its own vitality. That elastic outer layer thus inflated gives the relaxed-but-alive body its shape. Unfortunately, modern practices tend to yield bodies devoid of self-awareness, and therefore unable to sense this intrinsic form. Furthermore, modern-body energy often oscillates wildly and widely between hard tension and formless collapse. And the subtle, powerful energy of a vital and relaxed body eludes its owner.

Is it surprising, therefore, that a small, maybe invisible, pulse of energy born at the body-center moving along a limb and causing it to rise, is seen as lifting that limb? Excess effort is so common in daily practice that it becomes difficult to discern any movement otherwise. One solution to this problem is in sensing or even pretending that muscles are entirely slack such that bones are doing all the moving. At least this device draws attention to energy at the heart of a limb and away from bulk or exterior muscles. The same principal of observation can be applied to the core of the whole body, and to any component.

Suppose you're standing in one leg; all the torso weight is in it. You place the other leg in front, flat-soled and empty of all but its own weight. Your intention is to move into the forward leg. How does one do this according to the center, so to speak? Not by thrusting the back or standing leg. That would engage the exterior effort-muscles to the likely exclusion of the inner substance of locomotion, the sinews. Instead, begin to release the rear leg so that you feel the energy or weight moving toward its toe-pad. Remember, there is a strategic imperative already in place: to move an upright body forward along the ground. That means horizontally at your body center. Not up. Not down.

You will feel weight arriving in the front-leg heel-pad in synchrony with it leaving the rear-leg heel-pad. As you continue releasing the rear leg, your torso will be taken forward until you feel yourself standing in the front leg. The rear leg is now empty and somewhat behind, but not jacked up off the ground (See Chapter 4). The whole process is analog in form, rather like siphoning fluid from back leg into front leg. Common stepping tends toward digital, with little use of the knee-hinge: two stick-like limbs swung from lifted hips.

Tai Chi stepping therefore condenses to a rolling process, as if our feet are caterpillar tracking, as on bulldozers. There are places in this process where you can check the inter-feet relationship. First, the weight is in the rear or standing whole-foot, balanced front-to-back between heel-pad and toe-pad. Then as you begin releasing or flexing the rear leg, you are guided by the need to move horizontally; the center does not sink. The energy or weight will ease toward the toe-pad, and the front foot will become slightly weighted at its rear edge. Remember that this foot is softly flat on the ground. Next the front-foot heel-pad will engage as energy moves along the rear foot into its toe-pad and out of its heel-pad. Then you will feel the rear-foot toe-pad at its front edge synchronously with the front-foot heel-pad and rear part of its toe-pad. Finally, the weight will equalize in the front-foot heal-pad and toe-pad.

This process, which can be invisibly fast, merely requires reducing the difference between two limbs. There is greater stability around the stage when the two limbs are even-weighted and most alike. This is something to do with Central Equilibrium, one of five quintessential placements in Tai Chi Chuan (and little to do with dogma on double-weighted-ness). When two limbs have similar structure and energy, they can exchange form and purpose very efficiently, that is, seamlessly. This illustrates what is almost always missed, that Yin and Yang are joined, and interchange mostly in middle ground. In other words, there is only yin-ness and yang-ness usually exchanging smoothly about the centers of life processes, including locomotion.

Thus limbs with similar forms are to be preferred over those which are quite different, as in low postures wherein one leg is sharply angled and the other virtually straight. Such structures aren't useful if you need to move fluidly. This is apparent in ready-stances of many boxing styles, in sword-dueling, stalking, climbing, and tightrope-walking. All of these activities demand competence rather than show. Also, the skilled seem usually to be doing very little; there are only small changes between events, yet there is an admirable result overall.

The principle of similar limbs can be very helpful internally. It is not obvious that a fully weighted leg should have the same energetic guidelines as, say, a pendent arm. But releasing energy, though not structure, from the leg with the aim of matching its feel with that of the arm, is a very useful device. Effortless legs fulfill intent timelessly and seamlessly, no matter the purpose. And the same process of relating a tense part of the body to a relaxed part, offers an internal teacher always on-call. The eventual result is internal consistency, a homogeneity which can be sensed and maintained throughout Tai Chi practice.

So similar limbs really express an internal one-ness that most of us seek or wonder about. Arms usually get much more attention than legs. That's one of the problems. A main reason for this is that hands are at the ends of them, and hands tend to hog our attention, tool-users that we are. One lesson we can derive from this is that most of what we do with our hands requires arms that are reasonably flexed, moving in their mid-range (See Chapter 3). And the elbows vary in their hinging, as do the joints in the fingers. Tightly-closed joints anywhere become uncomfortable, because flow is reduced and yin-ness and yang-ness are much less able to relate. The same applies to fully extended arms, which merely become tired and would prefer to return toward the center.

The acquired illusion that our hands do most things can cause us to ignore the nature of the arms in general. Hands are merely ends of arms, and are quite far from the center. So reaching and grasping can induce inappropriate arm and body structures which are tiring or otherwise less than optimal. By centering attention closer to the arm centers, nearer elbows than hands, we can retain the important principle of option in movement. Running out of options in an engagement, means losing an advantage. Is this not forgetting Tai Chi Chuan?

The Tai Chi Classics address this when they say, All joints are rounded; and, All moves shall be comfortable. I would add, Energy moves fluently through a homogeneous medium and between matching structures or shapes. Mobile fluid moving through a straight tube (except a very small-bore one) loses less energy to friction than in any other shape. It is virtually free-flowing. Connect this straight tube to one with a right-angled bend, and flow is dramatically compromised. Cornering takes energy, as does increased eddying in the fluid. Flow is more lumpy, acquiring a more digital quality at the expense of smooth analog motion. Also, the corner causes backing-up; mismatching shapes thus influence flow at a distance from the problem.

This interruption or damping of flow will manifest, but less, if the added tube is curved, rather than angled. And if we now start with a curved tube, adding a straight one, flow will be similarly compromised. In either case, straight or curved, there is less interruption to original flow when adding a similar tube, straight to straight or curved to curved.

Human limbs are in general curved; the joints are rounded. These tubes, torso and limbs, transport a lot of fluid in all directions. And if our bodily pathways are similar curved tubes, so to speak, they can relate and exchange mass and energy easily. Why should it be otherwise? Thus two shallow-curved arms relate better than one shallow-curved and one sharply-curved. The shape or posture Holding-the-ball neatly illustrates a shallow curve in the pendent lower arm, and a sharp curve in the shoulder-level flexed arm. While this structure or process is useful, in application it would have come about in response to external events. In other words, the large difference between the shapes of your arms merely reflects counter-moves (and disadvantages in an opponent's situation).

Before Hold-the-ball took shape, your arms would likely have been in a combat-ready form like Raise hands. Here, the arms are complementary and curved to a similar degree. (However, it is also core practice in Tai Chi engagement to signal nothing, to merely wait devoid of extrinsic intent) Even in apparently large forms such as Diagonal flying or White crane spreads wings, only part of the process can be found in what the hands are doing and how far apart they are. In the former move, for example, the penetrating quality of the forward arm's energy may well bring the upper-arm or even the shoulder into contact. The rear arm may also engage close to its middle. The ensuing action would in effect apply two short limbs (the upper-arms) modestly close to the torso, despite the appearance of two hands well separated by elevation and distance. Similar limbs.

Initial practice in Tai Chi solo form resides in physical and structural exploration. Partner-practice dwells more in learning and harnessing the energies. Large energy differences between places of your contact on another body are less viable than a delicate balance. And exotic limb-forms are also less desirable during manipulations. Also, it's much more satisfying to allow your partner to self-defeat, so that your input is minimal or even unknown to the other. This situation will most often arise when small amounts and differences of energy prevail. In other words, when limbs are closely similar. Flow and exchange are more amenable between like than between unlike. There is an advantage to you in being connected with an angular body or one with large energy differences across it.

There is, however, ample evidence of long, low stances in Tai Chi Chuan past and present. This is worth pondering because pelvic rotation is restricted increasingly by separating feet beyond a modest step or shoulder-width. Such forms are demanding and usually restricted to special purposes, such as calisthenics and demonstration. Low stances can train the legs (invading a modern tendency to a stand-offish relationship with lower limbs), and encourage fluency in the pelvic girdle's range and maneuverability.

The principle of similarity should apply even between the bodies of partners or opponents. They move, you move. Their limb does something, yours adheres and follows. If you are sensitive enough you can borrow their energy at the still point as Yin changes to Yang, and vice-versa. The energies are small and similar. A body comprising smooth forms is quieter than an angular one, Therefore the quieter body receives signals better and sooner. Yet your small signals remain undetected by your opponent until it's too late.

It's also interesting that hard sparring styles like Tae Kwon Do have evolved from deep, wide-footed postures to higher, more rounded ones. The quality of sparring has improved with this trend, according to judges I have consulted. In the same way, it seems notable that ready postures in every style of Tai Chi Chuan or other internal art comprise four moderately curved limbs emanating from a moderately curved torso.

6

SLING THE REAR KNEE
It needs both ends
And works both ways

It may seem obvious to say or write. It also sounds obvious and easy when a student says, Yes or Uh-huh; there's that hint of impatience bespeaking the obvious to anyone with even half a brain. But in practice it's anything but obvious, despite total intellectual understanding of the concept. The concept. This so-simple concept expressed in movement is also so simple. But that does not mean easy to do.

In other words, when your body-center is oriented in its intended direction, and you begin to move that way, the legs should point-and-go that **same way**. The legs must point that way; and they must move that way. The former merely asserts that the leg as a whole ought to support the general intent. The latter addresses the question, When is a leg moving wholly forward or in any intended direction? What is the point of orienting the leading edge of an implement in a direction other than that intended for the rest of it? The edge goes one way the knife another? Obviously not.

Now observe a number of examples of human locomotion, including Tai Chi stepping. Do you often see weighted legs expressing congruence with the overall direction? Or do you observe legs going one way, it seems, while the torso points elsewhere? What may be wrong in this scenario is

addressed in Chapter 2. Energy that enters or leaves a foot shou
the energy of the whole body.

So if you are in a bow-stance with an angled rear leg, it's c
back into that leg so long as the limb remains centered; the center-line is
maintained in the rear foot. What is not ok for the energy and the knee-
oint is for the weight to shift **across** the foot, laterally or diagonally. The
knee will not be flexing in these cases, it will be twisting or wrenching,
however mildly. In a bow-stance, half the energy or weight is centered in
an angled leg, and that weight increases as you move back into it. Stillness
at the center of the leg, action as it moves overall.

n these circumstances, moving back is merely a matter of flexing the
rear knee: letting it flex, as distinct from making it wrench (lever) or twist
screw).Nothing could be simpler, mainly because doing Tai Chi is much
easier than not doing it. And when it's time to move forward, you need
only to let down the rear knee so that the leg seems to roll forward and
down: whole foot, toe-pad, shank, knee, even thigh. Cheng Man-ching
called this peeling the foot, although the peeling was actually an
expression of the whole leg moving down rather like the front end of
caterpillar tracking. It's important that the rear, emptying leg suspends
tself from the hip, pivoting on its toe-pad in the process The leg may then
move forward into a front-stance, wherein its toe-pad rests on the ground
close to the front foot.

Most movements using articulating limbs engage the mid-range (Chapter
5), where it also happens to be easier to miss the beginnings of
misalignment. Small movements characteristic of close work also present
possible problems. A small error of structure won't register as an obvious
disadvantage. A demanding partner will sense this weakness, of course.
Also, the distractions of in-fighting can blind you a little to what exactly
you are doing.

Thrusting, pushing your knee upward, will soon be dealt with by your rtner/opponent because it is so easy to feel. And misaligned knees are anathema to successful maneuvering, and to smooth passage of yang pulses through the body. Deeply flexed structures like Snake creeps down ask you to first open the angle of the back leg to about 90 degrees from the front-leg direction. Nonetheless, letting the rear leg shorten through its center-line should be purely a matter of flexing the rear knee, so that you end up sitting over the rear foot. The diminishing angle between shank and ground indicates the knee flowing downward. A small misalignment in this maneuver can force heavy stress in the knee by twisting, or levering the leg forward, letting weight drift into the inside edge of the rear foot. The knee is a joint you need two hands to surround; it is not just the knee-cap.

Squatting whip is one of those moves in which many seem to have difficulty relaxing the front leg as the body moves down. This happens because of inability to adequately empty or release a leg. And this in turn engenders a straight, pushed-back knee, a similar process to thrusting. Pushing or collapsing a knee toward the ground is not the same as letting it sling or flex downward. One thing your may also notice is that the weight is not in the back leg where it belongs, but between two legs, one very flexed and the other very straight (Chapter 5). The dreaded phrase, double-weighting has some applications, and this is one of them.

The principle of softening the rear knee, along with the whole leg, can be very helpful in the back-and-fore of partner practice and other engagements. It doesn't mean that the rear leg never opens, that is straightens. Moving out of a leg, or leaping, clearly engages opening-leg mechanisms. But neither action involves thrusting, common in the back leg, or pushing back the knee in a front leg. This is a difficult principle for many students, because not-thrusting seems to defy explanation in conscious terms. But it is simply an example of the thinking-mind's close relationship with bulk muscles. Each is, after all, an expression of an organism's exterior realm. Letting a leg open to a greater length is more a matter for sinews and instinct, that is, for the body's internal realm.

When a leg is flexing to take body-weight, there is no need to think about it. Most people, even in the formal practice of Tai Chi moves, just let the limb flex. It does so itself, so to speak. New students may have to train to regain some of the flexibility of their infancy. It is as much a matter of flexibility as of strength. The notion and practice of thrusting is usually so deeply ingrained by adulthood that letting a leg open or lengthen without it is forgotten.

A pertinent device is practicing three-step turns in which both feet leave the ground. These turns are common in martial arts, especially in weapons forms. They may involve 180 or 360 degrees in formal practice, but any angle of turn in application. In the first case, for example, starting in a left-leg back-stance, one steps down into the right leg, letting it flex as for jumping. In this case let's assume a clockwise body rotation. Therefore the right foot will engage a yang turn on its heel so that the toe rotates outward. The weight enters through the heel-pad, into the whole foot, and out through the toe-pad in one smooth move. In other words, you will spin the body in the process so that you end up landing on the left foot via the toe-pad, since you are now facing 180 degrees from the original direction. However, allow your body-weight to move back through the left foot and into the right foot so that you are now standing in a right-foot back-stance.

Remember, you are not jumping out of the original left leg, but out of the leg that you are stepping into, the right one. You have to take a leap of faith because you must not think of using this right leg. You must just let it open. When students ask how I made the jump, I have to own up and tell them that I have no idea. I cannot, as it unfolds, consciously articulate the process to them. The reason for this is quite simple: it is not a conscious process, but an internal one not using muscles per se but sinews or instinctual mechanism. The more you try to jump, the less easy it will be to let the leg close and open of its own accord, so to speak. Consider the move as along the ground rather than up and down. That way, you will engage in a process more like ordinary walking; internalized mechanisms are responsible for this action.

It may be good to walk yourself through the sequence enough to realize its flow and its analog nature. And to ensure that each transfer of weight through a foot and between both engages a falling energy in each knee. When you've learned the 180-degree turn you can extend the practice to 360 degrees. In this case, and using the same starting leg (standing in the left one), you will end up in a right-leg front-stance, and in the original direction. In between, you will turn about 180 degrees via the heel-then-toe of the pivoting right foot. You will then finish the turn (another 180 degrees) on the pivoting left toe-pad, ending up in a right-foot front-stance. Again, let yourself down into the right leg without engaging in the prospect of jumping out of it. Have faith: your leg knows perfectly well how to open naturally; it merely needs to re-acquaint itself with the forgotten mechanism. The overall practice principle here might be, as Cheng Man-ching would say, Invest in loss. In other words let consciousness mind its own business for a while.

Not-thrusting lets the knee flex softly forward, regardless of the action. And the jumping practice merely illustrates the body's intrinsic elasticity (or sung). Compress a soft spring, then release it. What does it do? It opens. But only if you let it.

7

HORSE-STANCE METHOD
Looks like Shaolin
Forging technique and tissue

At first glance horse-stances might imply anathema to Tai Chi principles and practice. Punditry persists in its condemnation of two feet planted on the ground. What comes up especially is double-weighting and how carefully we're supposed to avoid it. Since apparent double-weighting riddles this training method, it may be worth scrutiny.

Double-weighting has several basic meanings. To bipedal humans it can easily mean not moving, not getting anywhere. Hence the practice of standing in one leg in readiness for action. When one means to be active but somehow, in error or through lack of attention, finds one leg stuck to the ground, overall intent and momentary structure are at odds; that too is double-weighting. Even developing a magnificent athletic body, and acquiring flawless solo technique, but showing a weakness in martial spirit, is double-weighting, perhaps the most telling of all.

Two hands doing the same job, when one is sufficient, is double-weighting, as is two legs similarly engaged. And between two forceful bodies, in direct confrontation or on impact, there is double-weighting. These more physical examples could lead one to assume that standing in two legs is out of place in Tai Chi Chuan, which might be described as a superior art of natural movement.

But this art is born out of stillness, in which its techniques are seated, so to speak. Wu Ji standing is the mother of all postures. And it is a horse-stance, a high one, perhaps, but still a stance with equal leg-weighting. So it is not the structure of a horse-stance that is the problem. It is much more a case of an energy that is disintegrative, either through divergence or opposition or both. Wu Ji horse-stance is one that de-emphasizes physical energy; that is one of its purposes. Similar observations can be made about many chi gung stances, wherein intra-foot weighting may change but inter-feet weighting does not.

The training method espoused here has general application, but seemed to develop as a small arena in which to cohere various initially separate skills. I don't doubt that many practicers in complex disciplines have evolved such personal methods. These methods help to connect the dots, especially for slow learners like me. Thus horse-stance method proved useful for body conditioning, releasing, grounding, uniting above with below, repetition, pelvic rotation, and synchrony. And when seated in the breath, the methods open a way to healthful use of single postures or short sequences. In this way they represent common ground between solo form and chi gung, refining both technique and body substance. Also, because the feet remain in place, these methods are examples of Tai Chi practice in the space of a few square feet, something many pundits refer to, but almost never explain.

Horse-stance practice is inherently intense: it lends itself well to the principle, one thing a thousand times. It is therefore important to establish correct basic structure: that which works, and to maintain it while moving. This is a simple undertaking though not an easy one. Wu Ji standing offers the quintessential structure. But for these active exercises the center is lowered and the feet separated more. Just how low and wide depends on ability to soften the pelvic girdle and legs while maintaining Tai Chi structure, and on the desired intensity of practice. Less intense postures lend themselves more to repetition, which is desirable at earlier stages of practice. What is considered reasonable leg flexure by a seasoned practicer may be out of range to beginners. But a useful device may be to stand in one leg so that the other leg can sit laterally, in structure, and with the sole relaxed flat on the ground at a separation of about one shoulder-width plus a foot-width. Even here, in this modest stance, you should leave room to let yourself down a little, or let the feet separate a little more. You will not then be working at the edge of your body.

Horse-stance method uses weight-shifting. It is neither necessary nor desirable to extend the range to 100% weighting, however. Weight separations of 60/40 and perhaps 70/30 are enough if not substantial. In general, shift until the heavy leg is vertical. The higher the ratio, the more you'll need to lower the center. This in turn asks for well-flexed knees and supple ankles: a heavy-leg thigh is near horizontal at 70/30, yet both feet must adhere evenly to the flat ground. And it is important to maintain even weighting within each foot about its center-line during all weight-shifting (Chapter 2). One thing that needs constant checking, it seems, is parallel legs, which most people can observe as parallel feet. What are or are not parallel feet can get stuck in exterior observation. It is important to use the center of the feet as in natural motion (Chapter 2), in all assessments of parallel. The feet would appear to be on tram-lines, but at some width as already described.

Single Ward-off, Grasp sparrow's tail, Brush knee, Repulse monkey, Cloud hands, and Lady at shuttles lend themselves readily to Horse-stance method. Raise hands (though maybe not Play the pipa), White crane spreads wings, Diagonal flying, and Deflect-parry-punch are more complex or more prone to error because of rotations throughout the body, which need to be both synchronous and just sufficient. Efforts to rotate the center can easily exceed themselves, leading to twisted legs wherein knees and feet have lost their alignment (Chapter 3). This excess twisting may well force feet from the parallel, as well as self-destroy the foundation on which all movements depend.

The guidelines in general, and outlines of specific procedures, presume simple foot-wear allowing natural use of the feet. Such foot-wear will be thin-soled and horizontal: no raised heel. And no arch-supports, because the arch of a foot **is** a support, and a very well evolved one. Otherwise each method observes the following:

1. Movement emanates from an arch comprising legs and pelvic girdle.
2. Nose and navel maintain alignment along the torso's forward cardinal; do not turn the head.
3. The pelvic center, the lower dantien, remains absolutely horizontal.
4. Knees, your knees, maintain their cardinal direction, that is, forward. This needs care during pelvic rotations, which means just about always. A good test of where the action is and is not, is conducted while kneeling. With an erect body moving over reasonably separated knees, turn the pelvic girdle each way, noting that the knees do not move. Get the feel of this, finding the inner form of the action, by repetition. Then stand and repeat the exercise, preserving the feel of loose pelvis, and soft but aligned legs. The knees will drift slightly with shifting, of course.
5. Both foot-soles remain flat on the ground as if your shoes were empty.
6. Basic rules of Tai Chi alignment apply throughout. To practice otherwise is to learn very well how to do something really useless.

Single Ward-off is an important move: something like it appears early in the repertoire of almost all internal boxing styles. External applications aside, we can realize its form from the inside outward. Thus shifting weight into, say, the left foot should find the center lowered enough to maintain both legs in loose flexure, and the pelvic girdle level. Loose or suspended does not mean collapsed; the body is vitally full (sung). If the shift is too small, there won't be enough center-movement with which to synchronize relatively large changes in arm form and placement. 60/40 is adequate for a start, and a vertical heavy leg is a viable guide.

As for the upper body, the outer, higher arm is placed just as if you were in a classic poetry-reading stance, with the book held, pages upward, as you read the text. In other words, the fore-arm is turned palm-upward. The whole arm is slung with the hand at about throat-level. Slung means that the elbow is not held up, but is more like the arm of a violin player, except that the fore-arm is not vertical. It slopes at an inter-cardinal angle viewed from front or back and from the side: it is really part of a spiral arcing from shoulder to finger-tips. Much as I admire Cheng Man-ching's contributions to Tai Chi Chuan evolution, I do not recommend his usual practice in solo form of presenting a limp wrist. This is a very good training device for softening arms. But in the general active practices of a natural human body, wrists are Tai Chi-straight. The arm as a whole is curved of course, and a straight Tai Chi wrist merely continues this shallow curve (described more in Chapter 5).

If you train your higher arm with the in-facing palm parallel to the torso's vertical axis you will lose much of its generality or versatility. Thus you will not be practicing Tai Chi Chuan. Also, a vertical palm in this context can invite a lifted elbow, another anomaly in Tai Chi practice. An elbow may rise but it is seldom if ever lifted. In Ward-off the energy is inflationary (peng) and therefore along or through the arm from shoulder to finger-tips. That is why the hand (the end of an arm) faces both upward and backward to equal degree. You will need coiling flexibility to rotate the fore-arm to this degree. It needs to be done: I've come across young arms that already have difficulty rotating the palm through 180 degrees.

Fingers, too, are straight in the same sense as are the wrists. Curled fingers are a sign of habitual shortening along the inside of the hands (See The Foundation). In Ward-off, the penetrative function is no less important than others, such as deflection or rotational impact or indeed Shoulder-stroke. So much for the higher, outer arm in Ward-off.

The other arm falls forward and down, but much more down than forward; in double-peng the converse is true. In Cheng's sequence, Ward-off is preceded by Hold-the-ball, in which case the falling arm begins its descent from a folded horizontal structure at shoulder level. The hand of this upper arm is centered opposite the torso's center-line, and is palm-down. This position evolves each time you coil the center over the weighted leg. In other words, the pelvic girdle will rotate slightly to the right when the weight is more (or fully, if that is your wish) in the right leg or to the left while in the left leg. This coiling is pivoting because the torso/body-center is not shifting through space. In other contexts this coiling may accompany or be described as closing or compressing.

So starting in this coiled position in the right leg, right arm uppermost, you will move toward and into the left leg. In the process your center will rotate (but not be consciously turned) to face exactly front or cardinal. Meanwhile, the higher arm will float down and forward (Avoid deliberately extending it), ending up in front of the right thigh. This suspended-but-connected arm will now be Tai Chi-straight. Basically, you can just let the hand float vertically downward because the torso's uncoiling will bring the arm forward with it.

Thus the hand of the rising arm ascends a virtual vertical, the torso's center-line, and the falling hand descends a more-or-less true vertical. These are convenient relationships that may help synchronize the move's various components. Then the whole process is repeated from the left side, starting with the torso coiling to the left as the arms move synchronously into Hold-the-ball. The weight-shift need not be exactly similar each time; you just want a similar degree of shift for each weight-change.

The lower body or foundation will therefore coil then shift (this latter move to the front does, of course, engender a shallow uncoiling), coil then shift, while the upper body synchronously engages in Hold-the-ball then Ward-off, Hold-the-ball then Ward-off. Breathing is diaphragmic and through the nose. It may take many repetitions to establish synchrony or seamless changes. When you have attained high repeatability in the action you can re-check overall relaxation; tight spots can appear seemingly from nowhere. It is better to do a few tens of reps at a time before engaging in long sessions, wherein the number of reps loses itself in the slow blur of time merely passing. Practice correctly under these conditions. Who wants to acquire useless habits?

This is especially important when seating a movement in the breath. Poor matching of action with breath can induce internal scattering. You should not make the breath follow some intellectually contrived sequence of exercise, a typical human habit. When the diaphragm contracts, and sometimes the inter-costals with it, air flows into the body, which must yield to this prerogative. The organism as a whole may sometimes do something else, but that is another matter. Such processes are occasional to serve special purposes. Otherwise, and in this sequence of Ward-off, air leaves the body when the interior get smaller, and vice versa. Thus in Ward-off, coiling the torso over one of the legs, and synchronous fore-arm rotations in both arms as palms turn to face each other, plus folding of the upper arm, are together seated in the out-breath. As the exhalation ends, the body becomes maximally coiled. Neither process is compromised by force or tension. Similarly, uncoiling to the front and shifting to the other leg follow the in-breath. The Ward-off structure, actually a process of coordinated spirals, becomes fully realized as the in-breath reaches its elastic limit. And so on.

When all four limbs are coiled or folded to some degree, they are more densely packed, rather like a twisted towel. If the towel was initially saturated with water, it would clearly lose fluid as it was twisted and became more compact. That's just how one would wring out a towel. To where goes the fluid when that towel is represented by four coiling and folding limbs? Well, the human body is a more-or-less closed bag or membrane in which the most commonly used orifices are nose and mouth. In this context, these serve as access for air in and out of the lungs. Thus an exhalation is complemented by movement of fluids from the limbs (the periphery) into the torso; pressure increases while the diaphragm releases. We exhale. The circumference of the abdomen decreases in the process: hence the notion of belly or abdominal breathing. It is, of course, nothing of the kind; the diaphragm is the physical center of breathing.

Also, the body is relatively open and internally straight or uncoiled (despite an intrinsic braided structure of muscle systems) when it faces forward in Ward-off. The legs, too, face straight ahead with little active coiling in the thighs. Here the body is relatively open with a large internal volume, and this is a suitable vessel for inhalation. Internal metabolic oxygen consumption, and about 15 pounds/square inch of external atmosphere, don't really need much help when its time for an in-breath. That is why I consider inhalation as relaxation. And it may help explain Cheng's and his teacher's admonition to relax, relax, relax.

Moves such as Brush knee and Repulse monkey follow a pattern similar to Ward-off, coiling toward an inter-cardinal then shifting to another leg and facing cardinal. The intrinsic spiral of each component move covers the same degree of rotation. Coiling (or uncoiling) without shifting the body center or weight is tighter than coiling and shifting at the same time. Also, these rotations are what I would call front-stance rotations. In other words, if you step forward 100% in some move, such as Brush knee or Punch, your center will rotate from corner toward cardinal. Thus starting in a left-leg back-stance then moving forward into the right leg, your center will rotate clockwise until it reaches its natural limit oriented over the right leg toward the right inter-cardinal or corner. It will not reach a true inter-cardinal of 45 degrees from the right leg's orientation because the body's intrinsic structure will not permit it without force being applied. So a front-stance turn orients the center 20-to-30 degrees toward the outside of the standing limb, and anyway, much less than a back-stance rotation.

Back-stance angles are bigger than front-stance angles simply because the body is made that way; it seems so. The torso will naturally orient itself up to about 45 degrees to the standing leg in a back-stance. If the leg faces cardinal, then the center will point to the next inter-cardinal or corner. Thus a right-leg back-stance will find the leg oriented, say, north, and the torso facing north-west. The torso is well able to orient itself without force toward any intermediate angle; it just depends on the circumstances. The torso can also be persuaded (or forced) to point further west, something Cheng Man-ching asks you to do in Raise hands, Play the pipa, and White crane spreads wings. This is training just so long as the standing leg maintains its internal integrity and original orientation: that was Cheng's intention, I'm sure. Thereafter the leg is being twisted at the knee and lower: that is abuse.

When applying rotations in these Horse-stance methods it is therefore important to know what a relaxed rotation is, and when one reaches its limit. The front-stance turn is smaller and force will tend to make the leg bow outward, as the internal braiding tightens into hardness, pushing the knee out over the foot. The back-stance turn is bigger and looser, it seems. It is also more prone to over-rotation, dragging the knee inward so that the knee is pointing one way and the foot another. This is not just a case of knock-knees, but also of twisted knees, a double abuse. Trying to make a knee leave the center-line connecting hip, knee, and foot is counter to Tai Chi practice. Nonetheless, there are many instances of just this misalignment in Tai Chi iconography and visual aids. But I would say **never** let the knee move out of alignment with the rest of the leg, nor twist it so that it points in a direction other than exactly that of the foot's center-line (Chapter 2). There is not one iota of latitude in this rule of practice.

This may be difficult to remember in moves such as Raise hands and White crane. And perhaps more so in compound moves, such as Grasp sparrow's tail, in which there are mixtures of rotations, front-stance and back-stance. When Horse-stance method is applied to, say, Raise hands, the position of a completed move (arms have reached the peak of their outward flow) is when the torso will be oriented to the inter-cardinal, while the legs maintain their original cardinal direction. If you are seated in the left leg, the torso will face the right inter-cardinal, and vice versa. Thus the move ends up coiled rather than straight ahead, as in Ward-off. Mental effort-of-the-moment may induce a twisting attack on the standing knee. Also, discard any notion or action to thrust with the leg that you mean to empty. Thrusting with and emptying the same leg is a contradiction, that is, double-weighting. The light leg must be left to suspend from the hip while remaining connected, not collapsed (sung).

A forward angle in both upper-arms is essential to any action; vertical arms are characteristic of Wu Ji standing, the quintessentially still (externally inactive) structure. The arm over the standing leg in Raise hands is both closer to the body and lower than the other arm. This arm, over the light leg, may place the hand as high as the shoulders. In other words, the fore-arm of the light-side arm will slope upward. The lower arm over the standing leg will show a horizontal fore-arm, placing the hand at about solar-plexus level. (The energy is basically different if the fore-arm slopes down from the elbow) The overall arm structure is: one up-one down-one out-one back, in a form similar to many stances in martial arts.

The important practice of standing still in Raise hands may give the impression that the primary energy in the arms is one of, well, lifting. And this may well be a preoccupation early in long-term standing practice. Later, though, you may well find otherwise. What often saves you when the discomfort of suspended arms is intolerable is to direct your intent to energy **along** them. It's just like pointing with the digits except that there is no actual movement. This simple device is what you see when someone presents a putative unbendable arm for students or others to wrestle with (A flexed arm can be similarly unmovable, of course, as can any Tai Chi form).

This principle is important in practicing moves, like Raise hands, wherein the arms seem to be lifted. What is actually more important is that the arms are rising because energy is being directed along them. Energy is flowing out from the center, is it not? Blow into a sagging balloon and the structure will rise because of inflationary energy (peng). So it is with the arms, not only in Raise hands, but in any Tai Chi move in which energy moves out from the center. An active body, even when not moving, is filled with itself, a living and vital thing. And maintaining this fullness, like that of a moderately filled balloon, is what the whole body is doing when standing in, say, Raise hands. The overall energy is outward, and in Raise hands or other active structures, that energy moves along center-lines. Holding-up or lifting energy in a tube is almost counter or lateral to energy along the tube. Our arms are tubes. Our legs are tubes. Our torso is a tube.

White crane spreads wings uses this center-line energy (distinct from the center-line of the foot, Chapter 2) when an arm rises above its shoulder. Here, the upper-arm is oriented at about 45 degrees to the line joining both shoulders. It is also horizontal, placing the elbow level with the shoulder. It could be higher but it doesn't need to be for this example. Thus the fore-arm rises at an angle such that the back of the hand is about level and aligned with the torso's central axis. If you are still or stuck, lifting energy may first prevail. Later, the sense of energy along the arm takes over. So even in this edge-of-body technique when it seems that you must be lifting the arms, you are not. Hence my suggestion: limbs may rise but you don't need to lift them.

This whole explanation (Tai Chi Chuan is easier done than said) outlines basics for practice of repetitions, one of the main tools in Horse-stance methods. Repetition is worse than useless unless you are doing what you mean to do, and with an improving degree of repeatability. Each move need only be one that works, is classically "correct." And coiling into legs or a leg is a move that so easily gets overdone. That's where most so-called knee problems arise, in forcing knees out of alignment with the rest of the leg (or forcing torso-weight and ground-energy to double-weight into the front of a leg at the knee-joint).

Standing in a horse-stance without intent orients the torso and the whole body to the front cardinal. When you have shifted to one leg into a virtual back-stance (the light foot still adhering to the ground), you need to be oriented to the corner. In the right leg, you are facing the left corner, and vice versa. However, when you arrive at this angle it is important not to twist into it but to relax into it, and not collapse into it. Yes, the body turns in the move but you don't have to twist the torso-leg continuum to achieve this. So despite the concept of turning, stepping into a back-stance is as much straight as it is round. (Imagine you are backing into a typical parallel-sided parking slot. Your vehicle will be at some angle to the final orientation, so you have to turn the wheel to arc into the space. As you get closer to your resting place you need to adjust the curve of your path until it is virtually straight. Otherwise you're in danger of denting or clipping a couple of vehicles. Overall, you have ended up shifting from one straight to another straight, and there is a curve on the way. But that curve is only a means, not an end) So this is a case of the classical adage, In the round seek the straight.

The lower or falling arm in White crane floats down into the standard ready position of a suspended arm in front of the body (it is not collapsed), as in just prior to beginning the form, or at completion. In addition, the fore-arm is rotated outward orienting the palm at a right angle, maximum, to the torso's shoulder-line. In other words, each fore-arm (palm) rotates outward, one arm rising, the other falling. Sitting in this Horse-stance-method weighted leg is a virtual back-stance (It is virtual because usually the light front leg would move with and toward the rest of the body); the heavy-side arm will be up and vice-versa. The body-center is facing the corner and the fore-arms have rotated outward synchronously with the shift from center facing the cardinal. The center, equal weighted, position will find the fore-arms horizontal, and as if actually holding a ball: a soccer ball will do for size. The palms are vertical, and the upper-arms are sloping forward. From here you merely shift to the other leg, yielding the pattern: right back-stance, center horse-stance, left back-stance, and so on.

Again, if working in the breath, a White-crane stance will peak with an out-breath, and the hold-a-ball horse-stance will center at the limit of the in-breath. This only applies when you have achieved overall synchrony in the method. Movement must follow or adhere to the breath, and it must be your breath, not anyone else's. Each in- or out-breath need not be to full capacity; in which case you will eventually have to detach from the breath and let air and body go their own natural ways for a while.

How many repetitions? If the moves are synchronous and correct according to core Tai Chi principles, then practice until your are comfortably tired. Some can handle just a few minutes initially, and that may be good. Then you can loosen down a little before returning to the next session. The intensity of the practice should manifest in the repetitions, not in the physical discomfort of trying too hard. I preferred not to count at all but to set a timer somewhere at a distance for whatever period I sensed I could manage. That period can be an hour at a time for each technique. But what is the use of meaning to practice in the moment when your intent is locked onto some distant and maybe unrealistic target? Feel your way, and adhere to your common sense.

Horse-stance method also works well with short sets, such as Deflect-parry-punch. This is a three-component set which you must practice with a two-component (bipedal) body. The connecting move in my method is to shift from the cardinal punch in one leg to both arms slapping down palms-in to the corner outside the other leg. Therefore left-leg, right-arm punch to the cardinal (front) moves to both arms suspended in front of the right leg with the torso facing right (like a front-stance turn previously described). From there, you rotate the torso to the left corner without shifting, letting the arms fly into Deflect, also oriented to the left corner. Maintain your orientation, more or less, as you shift into the left leg for Parry (You can't really adopt an inside-leg or back-stance angle of 45 degrees in a front-stance turn; this will be more like 30 degrees. Just don't turn away from the leg you're moving into). Then shift into the right leg again for a left-arm Punch to the cardinal. And so on.

A three-move set is the longest sequence I care to practice as a single technique. Although at Tai Chi Chuan's shortest time-scale a skilled practicer can deliver several events per second, I prefer to limit internalization of **fast** sequences to three events. Otherwise there is the problem of engaging in a particular sequence when changing events call for something else. There is also an issue of pulse dynamics in an elastic (sung) body that is beyond the scope of these chapters. Suffice it to say here that it is a matter of singular intent and its corollary, recoil. The main issues in these methods are listed above. Short-term phenomena, such as repetitions, need to remain connected with Tai Chi Chuan's general practices, just as long forms need to be statements of invisibly short moments, if they are to maintain their integrity over time.

8

MISREADING ORIENTATION
It depends on your point of view
On target in all directions

Are you interested in applications of Tai Chi Chuan? Then don't be fooled by direction or big direction changes in a solo form. A serial of moves in a training set should suggest priorities and increasing levels of skill. But except for fundamentals laid out in the first few steps, it doesn't matter whether you face N, S, E, or West. And changing from one direction to another has little to do with applying moves in Tai Chi Chuan (boxing). Although the sequence of a form in any style is a programming device, applying postures in free-style exchanges has no sure sequence. Postures in action are processes.

Placing feet, and bodily rotations, are certainly key factors in developing agility and ability, and in managing internal energy. And forms address these subjects in a variety of ways, including formal direction changes. But when boxing or partner-practice is the focus, there seems to be a pre-eminent direction in Tai Chi Chuan. And that is toward your partner's or adversary's center. Any other orientation is an intended set-up, feint, or neutralization; or an invitation to defeat. In use, a 180-degree change between form postures could become 170, 17, or even 1.7 degrees. It merely depends on your instinctual intention and where you place your feet at any instant, which in turn depend on momentary unfolding events.

Solo form practice does train martial skills and other types of self-preservation. Tai Chi Chuan aims to keep you healthy under any circumstances and with decisive economy. Tai Chi Chuan can also be understood as an art of natural movement and as a window on or doorway to understanding strategy. Economy is the key and the principle. What things mean in Tai Chi Chuan is a matter of what is complementary: both/and, rather than what is exclusive: either/or.

Slow relaxed practice of integrated motion sharpens integral reflexes. Thus one's ability to do what humans are designed to do, place the body in one leg then another, is enhanced. We become more nimble. This applies to shifting, and to rotating, which are integral components of natural stepping, and of effective boxing and other engagements. These two basic means of moving our center, that is, our person, employ linear and circular principles respectively. In other words, they are aspects of classical straight and round.

And how is all this useful? Simply in joining knowing with doing. Cheng Man-ching's form opens in such a way as to illustrate these principles. First the center moves down then up; there is no shifting from the initial center-weighting. The arms rise as the center moves down. What lifts them? Not muscular power, because the Classics and every teacher keep saying: Relax, to which I would add: within structure. That is, it has little to do with conscious physical power. The form suggests: sink your total body-weight into the foot-centers and something will manifest, something that eludes and obviates conscious physical energy. It is, of course, intrinsic energy, whose tendency to flow increases as muscular force decreases.

The implication of Cheng's opener hints at allowing natural energy to flow, as distinct from doing something physical. Hence: Do It, don't do it, wherein It (intrinsic) and it (conscious effort) are distinguished. The fact that this lesson is at the beginning implies its application in all subsequent moves; that means principle. And because a form of increasing difficulty follows, it indicates the conditioning necessary to achieve the implied melding of energy and movement.

Since physical effort tends to inhibit intrinsic flow, we must be careful not to overdo things like twisting, in our enthusiasm to succeed. Allowing the center to move down expresses the direction down. Can this intent be overdone? Well yes, because the vertical torso can only remain so for a limited distance while both legs bear equal weight. Any lower, without canting-not-leaning, and the body will fall over backward, or at least will move toward the heel-pads. There is nothing wrong with varying the torso's heavenly orientation or its attitude to lines of gravity. However, how low your center is throughout the form is a matter of strategy, that elevation must be maintained unless you mean specifically otherwise. If you overdo it your legs will be unable to conform to the requirements of the center, which in this case means a smooth horizontal trajectory.

What you may notice as you shift into the left leg (which is what Cheng's form requires), is that the center can now go lower than it could at the limit of the initial horse-stance. That, though, is not the point at this juncture; but it can be a reminder to maintain elevation. What may be more important here is the principle of standing in one leg. And whereas two legs may offer an easier foundation, one leg demands to be used to the best of its ability. Thus the question arises: Best of its ability? One thing is certain, the torso can rotate readily in either direction, right or left. Cheng shifts us into the left foot.

As it empties, the right leg will exert a right-turning tendency. In other words, you'll find yourself sitting in a left back-stance with the right leg resting on the heel. This is a yang front leg because the lowering center causes the right knee to flex forward as it follows the center's inflationary or peng energy. Were you already at a low elevation, moving into a back-stance would tend to engage the right foot on its toe-pad. A relaxed back-stance will orient the torso at about 45 degrees to the weighted leg. That's a maximum angle for general purposes. This angle does not need any help from twisting the torso at the pelvic girdle, wherein lies the center. The structure is natural and habitual. Efforts to turn to a specific direction or through some fixed number of degrees can lead to force and forced-out structures in the weighted leg. The invitation here could be to know just what is an internally coiled, flexed leg, and what it feels like. Then if you must crank the torso through a larger angle, you will have the foundation of a classically comfortable leg on which to do it (See Chapter 3).

The opening of the solo form has so far said, lower the center strategically, shift the weight to one leg, and allow the torso to orient itself according to the foundation's structure. This hint at shifting to one side while turning toward the other is also tactics-via-strategy. If we assume an attack to your center it makes more sense to step to one side (say left) and turn toward the other. Not only have you evaded the straight attack with a round response, you will also find your opponent contained by your remaining three empty limbs. Empty limbs are competent limbs. Had you allowed the body to shift into the left while turning left, you may still have evaded the attack, but you will not be oriented toward your attacker. And you will be close to presenting your back via your right shoulder. Furthermore, your left arm will be on the left side of your torso and away from the line joining the two body-centers. These observations do not in any way preclude openness in your tactics. Rather, they express priorities in saving yourself and responding decisively, two principles melded in one action. If you always evade-and-attack as a single priority, or attack-and-evade, you will be expressing Tai Chi principles of engagement rather than something you might think up.

So the source of an attack also indicates a cardinal direction; you move toward this, evading as you do so. Cardinal, in turn, suggests corner or inter-cardinal, but there is no need to pivot the body specifically to achieve this orientation. The responding technique has the turn built into it. In other words, you evade the straight attack by not being where it would land. If you step back or move away, your body may alter its orientation in the process, but you may find that you are not facing your attacker's central axis. And you will have created more space between the two bodies, instead of less. That's what I call defending-defending; almost always you'll need to defend-attack.

If your attacker lunges in, then you may need only to shift, pivot, or step in to a small degree. This is because the force of the attack delivers the opponent into the zone most convenient for your counter. More usually, there will be a melding of the energies such that the two bodies join rather as would two dancers'. This is no dance, however. Your action will be moderate and enough to close the distance to your demonstrable advantage. In this case you will find yourself at some inter-cardinal angle to the attack and oriented toward your attacker's center (a new cardinal).

If you have turned your body too much, rather than let the tactic orient it, you will be vulnerable. This is because you have in effect begun to turn away from the source of the attack. An angle of 45 degrees is pretty close to ideal. If the attack is from S to N, say, then your response position will face SW or SE, and your will be pointing at the attacker's center. This doesn't mean that your front will be four-square toward the attacker, but that your instinct-intent will manifest that way. You could be countering with anything from a simple penetration with a single digit, to uprooting with a general torso-stroke. It just depends on the unfolding action. No matter what transpires, you must maintain the advantage gained from your initial counter. This advantage must be felt as a disadvantage by the opponent. And they must keep feeling it no matter what they do to counter or escape. That means the situation for the attacker is deteriorating. If Tai Chi principles apply, the attacking body will usually discombobulate itself through one or more spirals. This is because your orientation is sufficient to respond to the changes **and** to maintain the advantage, no more, no less. I summarize this as in-In-IN. Three should suffice; if not, you'll need to escape soon, because you may be out of your depth. Benign practice is another matter, of course.

Round-house attacks represent the other main component in Tai Chi maneuvers, the round. Here, the approach by an attacker is to your corner or inter-cardinal. This type of attack can be as far round as your lateral cardinal, that is, the shoulder-line. For two people nose-to-nose, so to speak, the primary cardinal is the line connecting the body-centers. This is the trajectory of straight-on attacks I've just sketched out. In countering a round-house as a maneuver, both bodies tend to rotate about a common center, as if they are standing on the rim of the wheel. As an arcing limb approaches, say, your left corner/side, you will step forward with your right side; the bodies become parallel again. Other moves can be made, such as a duck or cant, but this maneuver has a high priority at time-scales exceeding a half-second or so.

Your move should also close the distance so that you are in contact with a strategic advantage. This degree of contact would usually topple a partner if you inflated your body a little. Another way of viewing this type of contact is that your partner, assuming that you are training, rather than fighting, will feel slightly off-balance as you make contact. This situation shows up readily in a successful counter to a round-house attack because you will be inside your opponent's arms. Thus he/she will be on both heels, a no-no position in Tai Chi maneuvering, as you penetrate toward their center.

Someone standing in a post-holding or tree-hugging posture will indicate the basic body structure of many round-house attackers. So their second arm is an issue. But this is readily addressed because your left arm deals with the approaching right attack, and your right will end up inside the attacker's left. Again, the bodies move as if dancing together: a right-arm attack either misses your yielding left or is evaded as your move in with your right side. And vice versa. In any case, your counter-move will comprise an essentially straight move toward your opponent's in-arcing body.

You may end the attack right there. As the attacking limb comes around the circle, you respond along the radius of the same circle. Distance is time, after all, and here a quarter-second is worth more than a half-second. More commonly though, there will be a change in orientation by both bodies as you move to complement both the direction and orientation of the attack. And here again it is important not to twist your body or turn too much. You should end up emitting energy along a line that is essentially straight through you opponent's center (You may also attack the other's center by striking a vulnerable gate at another part of the body, but that's another matter for now). If you retrace or go over the event you will notice that a change in orientation from cardinal to inter-cardinal seldom needs to exceed 45 degrees. This rotation is a maximum in general practice, and is often less or much less.

It is very difficult to see or otherwise sense the shifts and turns of a skilled Tai Chi fighter. That is why many are led to express Tai Chi skill in hyperbole. Well, it isn't amazing. It's what a natural body can do. What is amazing, perhaps, is how much practice such good practicers have undergone to achieve that degree of invisibility. What kind of martial art is Tai Chi Chuan? The invisible kind. It's taken as a joke, but the joke is that it isn't one.

So big form-moves have their purpose: to train something. What is also important is that eventually Tai Chi principles are internalized. This means nothing less than re-acquiring your natural body. In such as organism, excess and deficiency are boundaries to natural dynamic equilibrium. The enthusiasm of practice plus old un-useful habits often thrust trainees into excessive movements instead of effective ones. The resilient, elastic interior of a natural body or, we hope, a Tai Chi body, keeps us near the center of ourselves. It's what might be called, maintenance of Yin. An attack on our person is expressing Yang; hence the Tai Chi adage, Let the other person attack first. Then you can read what they reveal.

A measured, practiced, response incorporates moderate movements. Over-doing is no better nor worse than under-doing. And a competent front step or stance includes the viability of rotation in either direction.

For a forward move from right leg to left leg this rotation may be up to about 30 degrees to the left: that's a front-stance turn. Usually the body will then reflex somewhat toward the right. The same step can engender a turn to the right. This turn is intrinsically larger at up to 45 degrees, and is characteristic of back-stances. Thus an even-weighted bow-stance works as if it is both front-stance and back-stance, because that is its potential in its center-position.

Similar principles of orientation apply to turning limbs. If you maintain centered limbs and optimally-open joints (two ways of saying the same thing), then a rotating palm or whatever can deliver whole-body energy. Since Tai Chi energy tends to be emitted in pulses, it follows that inner coiling of the body's substance needs to be just sufficient in degree and duration. Insistent coiling and rotations are to train the limits, to open the body so that it is useful right out to its edges. But to break structure in the effort is to self-destroy the foundation.

Inner scrutiny of body movement may well lead one to summarize muscles as a braided structure enclosing the bones. Unlike a simple braid of a shielded electrical cable, there seem to be many overlapping muscle and sinew braids all coiling among each other interdependently. This sense of inner structure comes not from pictures but from sensing internally how you and others move, be it freely or interrupted by tension. It's a kind of comparative body dynamics, which, in a natural or loose body is akin to fluid dynamics: liquid moving through and among protoplasmic tubing and tissue. Such descriptions seem bizarre even when one knows what one means, because there is something simply obvious about sensing natural movement. But is it easy?

Initial sensing of internal dynamics is like trying to read someone's thoughts. And the body-mind, which may be called the Mind or wisdom-mind or instinctual knowledge, is much more complex than the thinking-mind. So it may take patience, or rather, perseverance, to feel out your own internal workings.

Arms are much more accessible to early scrutiny than the legs on which we stand; at least the arms can hang relaxed with relative ease. Yet they can move too freely at times, rendering a collapsed structure. It is important to sense the ability of different parts of the arm to coil and hinge to different degrees (Chapter 3). And for accurate energy management it is very important to exercise only adequate energy. Otherwise there are going to be errors of direction and orientation and of excess and deficiency.

A common example of all these can manifest in a simple suspended arm. First, this arm is not collapsed; it is curved and springy along its length. If someone were to pull down gently on a suspended Tai Chi arm, and then release it, the arm would oscillate as does a light spring following extension and release. That's one reason why a hand will continue moving outward after the center itself has stopped moving. Second, the connection of the arm with the shoulder is open via a small rotation of the upper-arm, such that the palm faces back. This is merely the structure of two tubes linked so as to maintain optimum mutual flow. Some Tai Chi and Chinese medical texts refer to the joints as gates; these are best left open for whole-body work. I would add, seemingly redundantly, that the shoulder (or any) joint is never allowed to collapse without intent. Opening the arm's main connection to the torso is foundational Tai Chi practice.

The problem addressed here arises often in the lower arm of the simple structure, Hold-the-ball. The essential feature is that the fore-arm rotates, facing the palm forward-and-upward. The upper-arm remains still; the upper-arm does not rotate. Under these conditions a supple fore-arm will present a palm facing both forward and laterally. If you're facing S to start, the right palm before rotation will face N. When you've rotated the fore-arm the palm with face SE. If you end up with a S-facing palm, you have probably also rotated your upper-arm, collapsing or partially closing the shoulder-gate. This inadvertent closing of the arm's foundation is perhaps the most common structural error in arm movement.

What's happened is that the excess of trying to rotate the fore-arm has traveled up the arm, twisting the upper-arm. At the same time the shoulder has collapsed because of deficiency: it's such an easy-going joint. When the whole (right) arm remains connected, sung or springy-loose, the shoulder joint remains open and the palm will face the SE inter-cardinal. Clearly, if the inner orientations are in error, then the exterior ones are too. That invites defeat during engagement with a knowing partner/opponent. Also, such structures, while of no consequence in undemanding situations, can lead to physical injury when energy is high or invasion is forceful.

A body can be seen to be active when the upper-arms are forward of a vertical line below the arm-pits.. This is the line co-incident with the elbow at its lowest in a N-S trajectory (S-facing body); the elbow of a suspended arm moves in a curve with the shoulder at the curve's focus. An elbow can move behind this line, of course, but you just have to be careful. At its lowest point an elbow is at the back edge of a forward body, a place where it is less connected with humans' instinctual active direction, forward.

This limit is crucial when arms are relatively straight, and when they are high and out from the shoulder as in Single whip's hook-hand arm. Many students forget or don't realize that this position of the arm is closely related to action forward of and close to the body center. In some applications the inside of this extended arm's shoulder is attacking an opponent's body: an aspect of Shoulder-stroke or Torso-stroke. So it's important to maintain the arm's orientation within the body's intrinsic structure. An elbow may be viable behind the arm-pit line, but it is at the body's edge, so to speak. This in no way limits versatility, since it can be anywhere from across the front of the torso, to extended in front of the torso, to out at the side of the body, as in classical solo form. What is important is that the arm's orientation and the body's orientation are constrained by lines of intrinsic energy and structure.

Similar principles apply to flying legs, which are bigger, heavier, and thus more likely to exceed reasonable limits. The move often called Kick with heel is a fairly safe move in that the standing leg is as in a back-stance. But a common error is to twist the standing leg, the foundation of action in an effort to kick with the foot. A major component of this error is moving the leg with itself, instead of from the center. A good guide to viability is the classical, No part moves but the center moves first. Thus project the leg along its length and at an angle of 45 degrees maximum to the standing leg. In application, the two legs are often close to parallel. You are, after all, using the leg with exactly the same mechanism as when stepping forward in natural locomotion. This latter and Kick with heel use well-flexed knees, which can wave or flop. Orientation is less accurate from this shifty foundation.

To avoid errors in orientation the leg should be tossed out along its length by a small, springy rotation of the center. This is quite natural, since to start with, the limb is flexed, off the ground, with a horizontal thigh. As it de-flexes, it is merely getting longer because energy is moving along its length. The torso is virtually still when the foot reaches its peak height and distance (Anyway, the torso is no longer driving or pushing the leg; it has already sent its pulse). After the leg has reflexed the torso will end up oriented toward, but seldom at, the inter-cardinal from where it initiated the process. This description refers to full-speed better than to slow practice. A reflex is effortless; what is the point of pulling a spring that is compressed? It is redundant effort because you just need to let it re-open. Therefore, toss the leg out, then let it reflex. This property of a resilient body is intrinsic, and easily masked or overpowered by conscious effort.

One training device is to direct the flying leg toward a knee-high target. This inter-cardinal orientation (both forward and down) is close to the center of most applications. A flying heel level with its leg's hip-joint is at the top of the working range. Conducting a slow Kick with heel at this level with correct energy and structure is a challenge regardless of expertise. And a standing leg oriented at too big an angle from the target will often engender excess effort in the flying leg, and twisting at the foundation. It should be flying, not tortuously thrusting itself straight. Knees can be so easily abused during kicks, the standing knee because of twisting and the flying knee because of hinging and jacking into a virtual locked joint.

The same can be said with bells for Sweeping lotus leg, a Tai Chi-straight-legged move. The process is akin to swinging a long arm from pendent into a shoulder-high back-hand slap. The general application of Sweeping lotus leg is a lateral attack or counter; it's a corner or inter-cardinal technique. Basically, it delivers energy across the length-line of the flying leg, and is therefore not a pile-driving technique typical of hard-style practice. Also, there are many contact sites on the other body: it isn't just a kick. The end of the leg leaves the ground in a helical trajectory, getting as high as the body-center. If you incorporate lifting energy the leg can go higher. But really, what's the point? As for angular rotation, this can be a few degrees or even 45 degrees, the smaller angle applying more at closer range.

Projecting legs into targets, preferably firm-padded human ones, will show that smaller angles befit the pulse-like center-rotations that engender the action. Large angles, more than 45 degrees, dilute the explosive effect and increase the move's visibility. But they are ok for training. The same applies to Kick with heel, which is most useful at low elevations, small angles (typically 15 to 25 degrees), and close range. Training angles of close to 90 degrees are possible but the potential for internal twisting and wrenching increase sharply after about 45 degrees.

On the other hand, spins offer a large and practical rotational range, especially toe-pad spins. One can effectively turn through ¾-circle in practice, and more in training. A right-leg clockwise spin will orient you E for an attack from the S. That's not only a big change, it delivers a round response to a straight attack in accordance with Tai Chi principles (There are other tactical issues, such as back-turning, that are beyond the scope of this context).

In general, toe-spins offer a little more room in tight situations. A clockwise 45-degree right-foot toe-spin is useful for attacks to your right corner. And a 45-degree counter-clockwise turn deals with straight attacks; you can disappear and yet maintain a forward intent. If these attacks are sensed or countered earlier in their development, your spin will be smaller. The smaller turn is thus more decisive than a larger one. Testing changes in orientation indicates the value of economy. Smaller seems better in applications; larger changes make good training.

Heel-spins tend to take you more directly toward your partner/opponent, augmenting the intrinsic energy moving along the flying limb. Again, you'll notice that big changes in orientation actually detract from the move's effectiveness. One reason is that the rounder the energy form, the less straight the result. And the priority is to emit energy directly toward the other body's center. Therefore when your standing leg happens to be, say, 90 degrees from the target, you would need to spin on the heel to attain a viable orientation. Then you can emit from the smaller angle The whole process is a single movement, so there is no need to try emitting from a large angle. The larger orientation-change takes more time, and suggests a relatively large separation of bodies. Close work and small angles go together.

The solo form you learn should be a useful training device of principle and repertoire. But it is not a gospel. Neither are the words of your well-meaning instructor. Asking questions is a good approach, especially because Tai Chi forms include the obscure as well as the clear. So large orientation-changes in solo form can mislead and be misread. A careful study of small movements can be very revealing. And Tai Chi Chuan's seamless melding of intent and deed presents a veil to observers and opponents stuck in sensing only the exterior.

9

POWERS OF TEN

Faster! Slower!
Harnessing the fourth dimension

Whatever progress I have made in Tai Chi Chuan has developed on a foundation in other martial arts. These other disciplines offered firm stepping-stones in a quest to find a better way of doing something. Western boxing, knife-throwing, jujutsu, Five Animals, sword and staff, and especially Kuk Sool Won Hapkido comprise footings to essential basics. Progress has been cautious and slow, not because these arts were short on content, or because my only significant teacher, Yoo Jun-Saeng, lacked skill. Quite the contrary. So several decades of trying to learn something still find me deeply immersed in Tai Chi Chuan. Slow progress has, however, spawned a two-fold awareness of time. Such slow practice. Such a fast martial art.

Time-perception as a subject came up previously in a way that now connects with my Tai Chi practice. Even in my pre-teens knife-throwing, and in western boxing, time, at times, seemed almost to stand still. Some throws among hundreds moved in slow motion. They were the rare ones that I knew would land exactly on-target. In boxing, a similar process unfolded during some punches (not all mine), except that they replayed in slow motion after the event. This phenomenon became more frequent much later during Hapkido practice. A technique would emerge in the moment at a speed virtually invisible to an observer or recipient, but with apparent slowness in my replay of the event. It seemed like knowledge from nowhere; more likely the peaks and troughs in a naïve human's progress over uncharted terrain.

Tai Chi form practice evoked this sense of slow-motion, leading me early to trying moves at full speed. If Tai Chi Chuan was what some people said it was, then it seemed that it had to work at invisible speed. This invisibility is part in the techniques and part in the other person's senses. But I had not then discerned the mechanisms for this apparent speed in yang pulses and yin manipulations. My method was therefore to persist through a lot of trial and error. Large numbers of repetitions helped demonstrate body structures and dynamics that would have been less readily discerned at the usual slow pace of Tai Chi solo form practice.

It was rather like engaging in speed trials; things happen so fast you have no idea what you're doing. Basically, what took several seconds at a studied pace would take a fraction of a second in the time trial. I found two techniques helpful. One was staying as floppy as possible from the center up, but more or less maintaining overall poise and structure. This helped maintain alignments while applying a rag-doll feel of relaxation; in other words, edging close to collapse, while retaining some sense of body. Mindless repetition then mapped, inside and out, arm movements induced purely by throwing an arm (shoulder, elbow, wrist, fingers) with the center. In such moves, arm and shoulder remain loose, but they are also elastic. Elasticity is important. And it is important to discover where an arm goes for each pulse of the center.

It all starts in the unmoving foot-soles (See Chapter 2 and Chapter 8). These are the foundation for the whole leg/pelvic arch coiling and opening like a spring. Once this has begun you must let the rest of the body fulfill the shape engendered below. Do it, read it, try again; and without one iota of judgment about success or failure.

The second technique was to memorize with my body the places in space where the move arrives. For example, I wanted to locate the target area for the hand that rises slantingly upward in Ward-off. So for left Ward-off, I first adopt the finished bow-stance with my left hand opposite my nose-navel line and at the top of the torso. Next, I retrace the technique toward what came before, like reversing a movie sequence (which is not the move backward). In this case, the shape returned to is Hold-the-ball with the left hand at the bottom of the torso. Now I throw the arm/hand spirally upward with a pelvic pulse. The arm is loose, and the pulse is actually no more than an elastic 45-degree maximum rotation from the right inter-cardinal or SW toward the cardinal center at S. In essence, the feet and knees don't move. After the rotating pulse of the center or pelvic girdle, the torso will reflex back toward its starting position. This reflex never fully returns to its starting place. And it is important not to do anything to make it return or spring back. It is one move, not two: a rebound.

The overall picture is: sitting back in a S-facing bow-stance with the left leg in front. The arms are Holding-the-ball with the left arm below. The torso faces SW. As you move to the center of the bow-stance the arms exchange, the left rising and the right falling. The center/torso turns to S. Your left hand is now palm-in-and-up. It is not vertical; the fore-arm needs to maintain the rotation it uses to orient the palm upward in Hold-the-ball. The left hand arrives at about the elevation of the top of the torso or neck-height. The right arm, starting with wrist at shoulder-level, elbow flexed and slightly settled (not slung), falls from its place at the top of the torso. The whole arm opens as it floats down into a suspended palm-in Ready position. This right hand in essence falls vertically, despite the body as a whole moving through space.

As you repeat the exercise, a pattern or, rather, a design, will emerge. The point-destination of the flying left hand is something you can sense, even though there is nothing there in solo practice. If you try to figure out the movement intellectually, you'll no doubt find it to be just too complicated. Yet the process is a complex one. But by concentrating on repeating the simple aim of the exercise, to find where the hand arrives, you will engage the complexity internally as a body-move. Repetition needs checks of basics, such as firm lower legs, not thrusting into the bow-stance, keeping loose-and-springy (sung) arms, breathing naturally through the nose, an upright torso, and not letting the shank of the front (left) leg move through the vertical to end up sloping forward. The general form is a wedging back-hand to the air in front of you at the S cardinal. Its design mimics a twist-drill with the torso's vertical axis as the core, and the arm as the Archimedean cutter.

My own practice engendered a definite sense of moving through a three-dimensional shape in space. It's difficult to articulate accurately, but Ward-off felt rather like a spiral staircase; its axis my axis, and the hand-rail the trajectory of my rising left hand. One of the purposes of the exercise is to internalize the dynamic form of the move so that it becomes one thing, not several components (Understanding components is important, however). This form applies to Cheng Man-ching's (up) or Yang Lu-chan's (down) initial palm orientation in the lower arm. For me, the form began outside of my body, as something I could observe in a mirror (one reason why there are no mirrors in my training-hall). But it became something I did from inside, under the gaze of a spherical eye at my lower dantien. This experience was not like flicking a switch, more like a light coming on occasionally and then with increasing frequency, transforming from exception to usual.

It's important to keep checking basic structure so that tension and slackness don't intrude. Tightening then releasing, and firming deliberate slackness, are good tests of what these faults feel like. You must experiment and learn from your bodily sensations. At the outset it takes a lot of attention, but with repeated practice, this too internalizes. The stunning value of internalizing basics didn't hit me until later, a neat reminder of Cheng Man-ching's advice not to be greedy. The reward in this case is the ability to place your hand or arm or elbow or shoulder just where you need it without thinking and without apparent effort.

Eventually you should be able to deliver a hand full-speed to a small area, and with a range that discerns the thickness of a piece of paper. You can, of course, practice moves using an external target; feedback helps. But this has an external dimension eventually redundant in the interior realm. Furthermore, we have a faculty that senses from the inside exactly where our body is. You can locate fingers very accurately using their touch sensors. Well, you can do that from the inside; they are, after all, three-dimensional tissues, and there are millions of them throughout our organism. It is not amazing that a human can punch a piece of paper without punching the surface on which it is resting. Well, perhaps it is, just like the rest of Nature.

There are many moves throughout the form and many body-parts to observe. What you learn in principle from persistently studying one move will roll over into others. A period of speed practice is well served by complementary slow practice. Always come back to slow practice: that's where the principle of relaxation-without-collapse (sung) is always ready to teach just a little bit more. It will certainly remind persistent Tai Chi students that fast only seems fast to an external observer, in line with a Classical adage that all moves shall be comfortable.

It is not a huge leap from How fast? to How slow? But this question came to me much later than it should have. If you fall flat on your face once in a while, then you're making progress. This was my convenient reasoning anyway, when after a lot of practice, a certain penny dropped. I realized that some sports-people envisioned dry runs just before doing the real thing. And there was a jockey who walked the course before a race, not just to learn its topography and condition, but to visualize the more difficult maneuvers. Such previews of events are so common, in fact, that their significance is easy to miss, or so I excused myself. Also, Tai Chi practice is already so slow that the concept of slow-motion run-ups just didn't arise.

But eventually it did. And it proved really useful in action. Ultra-slow form neatly joined stillness and motion, standing and stepping. Slowing a sequence from, say, three seconds to 30, certainly revealed rusty joints, sticky tissues, and more general tension. It also gave a hundred opportunities to relax or release for each inch of movement. And the (then unknown) Classic aphorism, Learn the inches, then the hundredths...materialized into practice.

Ten times slower not only offers thousands of chances to relax and align in just a single weight-shift or rotation, it also helps co-ordinate different-sized movements in various parts of the body. A simple example is the right turn following right Ward-off or Double peng with the right leg forward. The legs remain exactly in a right bow-stance while the pelvic girdle rotates about 30 degrees from the cardinal to the right. Meanwhile, and in precise synchrony, the Ward-off arm (the right) rotates its fore-arm from palm-in-and-up to palm-down-and-out, a rotation of about 180 degrees. Precise synchrony in principal means that for each degree of rotation at the center, the fore-arm rotates nine degrees. In practice it may be better to relate, say, one-quarter completion of one movement with the same degree of change in the other. Thus about five degrees of rotation at the center corresponds to 45 degrees in the fore-arm. But any sense of two events unfolding in step is an advantage. It's rather like watching two different-sized cogs meshing in mutual rotation.

Other movements may change limb positions relative to the body center. For example, the left hand in Double peng, which sat palm-forward-and-down several inches inside the right hand, rotates to palm-up with the same pelvic-girdle rotation. At the same time, the left arm moves from in front of the central axis to across the front of the torso, placing the fore-arm horizontal with its hand palm-up just inside of the right elbow. So the left hand (as the upper-arm rotates and pivots at the shoulder) can travel about a foot in exact partnership with the other changes. Observing each change: rotating a fore-arm or moving a limb or part of it in concert with the change at the center, offers opportunities to co-ordinate each component of a move. Then you can sense the inter-dependence of each component with another component, sometimes in the same limb, as in the left fore-arm both rotating and moving through space. Or you can sense the relationship between two rotations in different limbs. Eventually, each change becomes joined to any other change that's taking part in the move (One part moves, all parts move, until single and plural condense). The center turns, an arm flies, the other rotates in the fore-arm. The center shifts without rotating, and the same limb changes may occur. And so on...

What's important is that they are all synchronous changes that slow scrutiny, observing each iota of change, helps to internalize. This is not usually a single event; internal pathways need to become re-established as effective beneficial devices. But getting a glimpse is good reason to recap and try again. Bear in mind that once something is internalized, like which digit is working which keys on a keyboard, backward as a concept tends to disappear. I'm not referring to the direction back. I mean whether a move is unfolding or refolding. Soon a technique works this way **and** that way. It is not a move being done backward. Thus you can co-ordinate a move and, importantly, part of a move (all Tai Chi movements have applications) first one way, then re-trace its structure toward its starting position. Moving slowly enough to realize the process **with your body**, is an invaluable tool in self-revelation. Speed comes soon enough. It never seems fast in the present to the performer: it just happens.

As you step through standard form practice, the overall shape of each move will become clearer. You must, of course, give each move time and relaxed scrutiny. This is important because at any time you're honing one thing, with eventual benefit to many. That's a significant step toward the intent becoming the deed, a relationship that transcends conscious awareness of time. Also, after practicing the ultra-slow method, regular form practice can develop an internal unctuous, oily feel. This, too, is a useful step toward seamless technique, something one never stops pursuing, like elastic relaxation (sung). And although it is not the issue during actuation, your understanding of what, exactly, is going on, can be helpful to others.

Something you may notice after extended slow-method practice is that joints and muscles can acquire a creaky, almost digital quality during their changes. My hands have felt as if they were made of concrete. My feeling about this is that intent, however benign, can be very powerful. And until the exterior body learns its true place in the proceedings, it will do its best to fulfill your intent. And since the moves are so slow, the afterglow of an effort in one instant can carry over into the next, eventually adding up to concrete, so to speak. This is an analog of a life-long tendency in many bodies to get tenser and harder, leading to disharmony, chronic stiffness, and sickness.

Therefore always engage in loosening-down (better than loosening-up) after any period of intense practice. This is especially important if you've been practicing leg moves that involve thighs becoming horizontal, whether that's because the leg is flying or because you're lowering the center. And finally, maintain natural diaphragmic breathing through the nose. Fast methods may engender breath patterns other than those you would normally expect from sedate movements. Let them be. But if you're holding breath at any time, something is wrong. It's a habit that's worth losing. In life, breath comes first and last, and meanwhile continues.

10

PERFECT BALANCE
Embrace gravity, return to center
Stop-frames and seamless texture

The word perfect, like master, should not qualify Tai Chi Chuan. Which student, after all, would mislead himself by expecting or accepting either? But it is a demanding word implying no details. Balance here refers to an internalized state rather than to an external parameter. Inquisition is a useful tool, but measurement becomes displaced by instinct, the one dependent on time and distance, the other independent of either. The very time taken to frame words, is an effective barrier to sensing the timelessness in applied Tai Chi practice. So although Perfect Balance may mean balanced at every instant, it isn't really sensed as a digital parameter. If you are balanced then you don't need to stop for measurement. You need merely to maintain what is already there. This better describes something seamless than something you keep doing, which is by nature digital. Tai Chi phenomena transcend the ability of words to describe them, one reason, perhaps, for poetic description.

But words can be useful to establish word-concepts as stepping-stones to experience in bodies. So Perfect Balance means feeling balanced at any moment you might choose to examine your state. A singular body-sense of perfect balance during solo-form practice is a good place to start. However, this sense can manifest anywhere, anytime, no matter what you are doing. It offers two rewards: a reliable constant at any moment, and a stepping-stone toward greater complexity. Every human begins engaging or learning about complexity with a marshalling of components, whether the subject is their own gestation, cosmology, or simply stepping with confidence across difficult terrain.

A beginner might engage with coordinating rotations in two parts of the body (There are parts initially) until they are truly interdependent and complementary (Chapters 3 and 9). A more skilled practicer might first establish or register a one-sense of something like balance or co-ordination, and then proceed to maintain that sense during movement (Chapter 1). Each pursues or engages some quality of continuity. And each in doing so moves toward generality in practice. For the relative beginner all this will be applied in solo practice. As experience mounts, these skills will be tested and refined by two-person practice.

Every move in the solo form, not just commonly recognized postures, addresses internal solo energy, and possible interplay of two or more bodies. The Classical adage that all moves shall be comfortable, basically acknowledges the principle of balance. And by saying that all moves should be such, the adage implies preserving that balance. So if Perfect Balance is one half of a zipper, then continuity is the other half. As soon as one half falters, there is opportunity for someone to interrupt the other. Postures per se disappear in dynamic application. Ward-off and other titles refer not so much to postures as to processes, not to position but to movement. What illustrates this is inventing self-defense scenarios and asking which Tai Chi posture would apply. New students tend to ponder the matter; more experienced ones will vote for any posture.

It is, of course, a trick question, a Tai Chi smile, so to speak. Any posture if enacted as process according to Tai Chi principles will employ relaxation, alignment, centering, et al, which is more useful than thinking about applications. What is needed is a comfortable, moving response that will re-balance a disharmony as it unfolds. One conserves internal uniformity in moving out of Wu Ji stillness. And one conserves Perfect Balance in active engagement with others. Thus solo-form practice guided by balance and continuity is excellent martial conditioning, whether or not that is the intention. In other words, it is unnecessary to practice solo form for a particular reason. The form's usefulness is as pervasive as the influence of gravity that monitors your balance.

It may seem strange, therefore, to apply digital movement to enhancing continuous balance. But this is what you can do to help align and release each inch of the way. The importance to balance of flat foot-soles (Chapter 2), a floating head, heavy knees and elbows, soft-and-open hands (The Foundation), and a soft, even floppy, abdomen, comes repeatedly under scrutiny. And the downward energy of releasing musculature offers a sense similar to that of flexing the knees and sinking the center. In other words, downward energy enhances balance, increasing stability.

Merely following whatever balance you may have either at the center (one aspect of sinking the chi to the lower dantien) or in the foot-soles also highlights sagging. Although sagging may seem less energetic, it also closes somewhat the interior pathways; internal energy flows less well. Distinguishing relaxing and collapsing is a long-term rewarding meditation; it is a pursuit of sung or elasticity.

Perfect balance becomes more critical as the body approaches its viable limits. Squatting whip (Snake creeps down) and Sweeping lotus leg are edge-of-the-body techniques in which balance is critical in application but often uncertain in solo form; and repeatedly so. Squatting whip maintains a vertical torso; there is no need to cant, which is a balanced-on-the-spot tilt of the torso. Learn the difference between canting and leaning. Canting maintains the position of the center; leaning moves it. The center, which here rotates vertically about the lower dantien, therefore stays balanced within the body. You can relax into this type of structure. Leaning requires extra energy to hold the body up. And, anyway, breathing into the center is compromised by leaning. So a floppy abdomen is not so much a device, more a component of a balanced body.

Lowering yourself into the back leg is not made easier by leaning the body, although it may offer that illusion. It merely lowers the upper-body (intent to get down) instead of doing the work where needed, in the upper-leg and hip. Thus the body twice doesn't do what it needs to: strengthen the legs, and maintain balance in a difficult move.

I have found that canting while moving back or down is readily open to exploitation by another person. Doing both can be disastrous even with an unskilled partner. At higher speeds, canting finds use as a dodge. And this dodge works at any orientation of the torso. Here, I refer to the center of balance, the lower dantien, as a universal joint. Although it doesn't exist in the terms of biomass, it is the most important joint in matters of acquiring and conserving balance. If the body is balanced around this point, then it is viable in all Tai Chi Chuan applications. Leaning in any form, to any degree, invades this dynamic integrity. The torso's central axis even when vertical is not geometrically straight. It is more like a fishing rod, whose core is aligned at any degree of flexure. Most torsos are not quite that flexible, but they may flex to some degree toward any point on the compass. So in canting it is important to maintain the integrity implied by the curve of a flexed-and-connected (sung) torso. Otherwise the best-intended cant is merely another act of leaning.

Backward canting is thus viable in a Tai Chi body; but has a low priority in Tai Chi maneuvering. One can, of course, exploit a tendency of the lower-body (that below the center) to move forward, but the intricacies of such maneuvers exceed the scope of this chapter.

Swinging legs is a similarly challenging subject. Perhaps one of the main components of sustained balance during leg moves is two relaxed limbs. There is no excess effort. The intention in standing or moving legs is that they be equally relaxed, despite the fullness of the standing one. Otherwise, the body-center or lower abdomen can get caught between, forming a stiff, unstable, angular structure. Balance is lost, the instability self-inflicted. One training device is a Tai Chi in-breath as the empty leg moves outward; it's difficult to do this with a contracted lower body. Another is to learn sensing the body-weight neatly balanced right down through the center of the standing limb. Also, you can try reducing the size of a move by using a smaller angle of rotation, or limiting the range of an outward-moving limb.

What motivates any moving leg is movement at and by the body-center. It is usually a smooth pulse, and frequently a rotation. And for training I would construe that rotation as 45 degrees maximum. In action this rotation is often much smaller. The success of the center's actuating pulse has much to do with an empty flying leg. And maintaining a comfortable, settled center is concomitant with the energy moving outward along the flying limb. I have found it good advice to invest in loss (Cheng Man-ching's aphorism), and find just where the center's pulse sends the empty leg, however many repetitions it takes. On the way, there is ample opportunity to maintain your balance and empty the flying limb.

Here are two further training devices. One is do not at first engage in slow kicks. Percussive energy is short-lived in application. And any limb may be delivering a pulse (Strikes tend to be more common with arms). So this type of leg-training lends itself to shorter time-scales (Chapter 9). When you have acquired reasonable fluency in the overall form of the move, you may find it fruitful gradually to slow the pace. Softening a slow-flying leg is an intriguing challenge. The other device may ease this process. It is to maintain the form and general intent of a desired move (like Kick with heel), while sending the flying foot to a lower destination. Too much effort can be applied or wasted over the short and long term in trying to kick something at waist height. This location, and even higher, can be part of training, but the overall energy of the move may be better understood by letting the foot (as the end of a leg) fall to standing-knee height. There are many applications even lower. No matter the intention it is the leg on the ground that places the flying one, via a calm, balanced center. Spectacular kicks can so easily make a spectacle of the would-be kicker.

Perfect Balance helps bring fluency to all Tai Chi practices. Learning postures is valuable for structure, endurance, and internal power, and to seat forms firmly in the instincts. Much difficulty seems to arise between postures, often described as transitional moves. Perfect Balance helps build bridges between better-known structures, eventually rendering the concept of transitional redundant. Using the body-center (lower dantien) as a fulcrum between front and rear, left and right, corner and corner, arm and arm, leg and leg, arm and leg, and so on, offers a one-sense of structure and aligned energy. You can apply this sense of balance in any situation merely by maintaining your attention or awareness there. This crux of the matter is no concept; experiment with your body.

It is ok, even necessary, to engage in unstructured competition, to experience unknown or green energy. But you should stop to investigate errors as they arise. Otherwise the crux, when, where, and how you left your center, will be overlooked. This happens a lot in partner practice. One person will topple or become tangled and that's the end of it; the process is ignored in the heat of the moment. Whenever things come to a stop or feel tight, it is time to take a look at why and when. Not to do so is to let force or error decide the structure of the practice. Partner-practice is two people learning no matter the skill of each. Slow down to a crawl, and pay attention to balance, simple and compound, in all directions. And repeat the troublesome event until you can prevent it from materializing. Both partners will then be engaged in the same process: learning to manipulate and apply less energy in shorter time spans. Balance maintained means seamless movement, in other words, Tai Chi Chuan.

THE PROSPECT / APPARENT CLOSURE

Why practice Tai Chi Chuan?
That's the second question

Can one learn Tai Chi Chuan from a book, with no teacher?
My answer is that this is a very good question.
—Cheng Man-ching (1901-1975)

Tai Chi Chuan is a human product and a product of many humans. In essence, it aims to neutralize any tendency that reduces the quality and duration of human life. Profound yet liberating, its premise is the ability of humans to evolve into superior beings. Evolve connotes improve. But how can one improve on evolution or creation, so to speak? Cheng neatly side-steps this issue by observing that he never wanted to become a Buddha; he merely wanted to become a man. For a master of five excellences (martial arts, medicine, poetry, calligraphy, and art) to say such a thing implies a boundless prospect in a quest of human complexity. That is enough, is it not?

In other words, what one human can to do is an exemplar for any human. The subject is not circumstances. It is an intrinsic ability of each human to ask about their part in the universe. This is a process of absorption and benevolent contemplation. Equally it is a process of application, of testing, without goal or judgment. Tai Chi Chuan is thus viable as a method of re-orienting oneself away from a fragmented modern body toward an integrated natural one. Structured training within the principles of Tai Chi Chuan offers sensing and embracing our human essence as a homologue of some greater design. Like any such discipline, secular or sacred, Tai

Chi practice invokes sooner or later a singular energy, structure, or entity, rather than many. The numbers should get smaller, and lists become redundant; attention begets sensitivity, information condenses to knowledge, and experience to instinct.

The integration that Tai Chi practice encourages renders the complication of fragmentary habits redundant. People and other beings in their natural (some might say God-given or primitive) state don't need Tai Chi Chuan; except maybe to play games. Life is above all a generality needing no separate special knowledge. And if there are ways to lessen the civilized tendency to grab the special at the expense of the general, one of those ways is Tai Chi Chuan.

The many who forged Tai Chi Chuan from its components, formulated something that distinguishes intelligence and intellect. Cerebration, though attractive, is a part, a minor attribute, of the whole organism; hence an understanding of intellect as distinct from intelligence. The Mandarin character for mind and heart is the same. This hints that the power of the intellect is most useful under the influence of the whole organism's greater complexity. This is the true repository of accumulated knowledge, deep instinct, and wisdom. Thus we can begin to appreciate the intrinsic attributes of humans in general, and even the dangers of unbridled intellect.

This is not high-flown theory but a practical matter in acquiring Tai Chi principles. It is surely useful to learn that stylists and masters are specialists, and redundant in the long run. Mastery in a martial art is just another horizon, an end of a rainbow. One needs to enjoy the walk rather than fix one's vision or expectation on an obvious illusion. A time comes when even a master must recoup and return from giving answers to asking questions. To improve, humans need merely to know themselves better, something anyone with a body can do. Tai Chi Chuan offers other strata of knowledge, as Cheng showed. But it is mainly a body-centered discipline.

That, surely, is the genius within this art. Simple (without saying easy) interest in our own organism, guided by gravity and economy, in stillness and in motion, offers a path toward wholeness. High intellect brings the horizon no closer, while simple steps do. Yet the quest maintains its feel-good factor. Any Tai chi student can be inspired on seeing a distant agile young practicer become a 90-year-old at close quarters.

Placing our feet on the ground with care, patience, and economy can enhance quantity and quality in our lives. This attractive prospect is shadowed by what our bodies have become over recent generations, and by what we do with them after birth. Each such body has its own relationship with natural movement. But through Tai Chi practice we let go these acquired differences, and progressively eliminate the turbid, allowing the clear to rise.

This important aphorism from classical Chinese medicine refers to digestive maturation of food into waste and nutrient. It resonates strongly with a process of human growth in general. The saying implies that personal maturation asks us to let go of what we don't need, and to distil or streamline what we do. Tai Chi Chuan embodies a close analog in relax or release excess energy, and align or improve structure and process. It's one principle and the other. It is not either/or.

These are not things to think about. They are things you allow or you intend to (will) do. A unique feature of Tai Chi practice is that it quiets the neurological system. Thought then becomes less intrusive simply by being less frequent. A calm, receptive thinking-mind allows and enhances patient scrutiny of what we feel. And constantly engaging with what's happening in our bodies doesn't allow much time to think. This and other known benefits of moving toward integrative self-sensing are too numerous to list here. Tai Chi therapy's role in general improvement and in alleviating many disharmonies is a matter of world-wide public record.

The principle of self-study implies clearly that no-one else can do it for you. Others may assist but if they are effective they eventually render themselves redundant. Each person has the inherent ability to try and succeed in Tai Chi Chuan. The aim is competence not foolish mastery. There are no side-effects to adequate practice. A form done 50% well yields 50% of the benefits. The methods presented here allow each person to improve from the center outward with little or no extrinsic assistance.

This may not be everyone's choice; self-learning is actually self-teaching. However, the methods can also augment learning from others. They enhance internal knowledge which smoothes the processes of absorption. And the methods tend to improve the quality of Tai Chi practice itself: an evolving future for an evolving body.

No one method is better than another in this series. And each person can exercise her or his preferences. They are spokes in the same wheel, so to speak, and it doesn't matter whether you approach the hub directly along one spoke, or spiral in along several. What initially may seem to be quite different devices, will emerge as ways of serving the center. The methods are convergent and complementary.

Tai Chi practice sooner or later impinges on the milieu of everyday life. Hewing wood and drawing water are equal and complementary to Tai Chi practice. Many useless habits are acquired, first in our seats of learning, and later in the work-place, as well as from modern culture. And it seems virtually impossible to re-integrate ourselves without first realizing an opposing tendency in modern life. Cheng Man-ching nodded to this tendency with the teasing observation that he practiced Tai Chi Chuan 24 hours a day.

However, there is no need to further fragment ourselves by chasing all possible errors. Everyone has a body, and this is a crucible for much learning and self-teaching. You can feel directly the useless and damaging constraints in modern footwear. Binding feet and heads may be over, but binding the body with elastic garments, sometimes several layers of them, is strongly in vogue. And belts that strangle the lower torso and its vital contents are all too common. Tai Chi practice enhances sensitivity to any invasion of the body's preferred state of relaxed fluidity (sung).

The Tai Chi skill of opening internal pathways for natural energy, highlights the discomfort of poor posture. Ingesting and digesting food and drink, your future-self, require the same bodily alignment as breathing air, our other main nutrient. And you may become increasingly aware of inhumane design in devices, utensils, and furniture in everyday use. Tai Chi Chuan could well be an apt source for the science of ergonomics; yet another story.

Breathing quietly through the nose is at the heart of most methods presented here, and of Tai Chi Chuan in general. Physical effort, conscious trying, is neither needed nor desired in Tai Chi breathing. It's gentleness harnesses air's natural pressure, which fills our lungs at 15lb per square inch. It is easier to let air in than to push it out, is it not? Air force is fluid and so is felt as something elastic rather than rigid. But it is powerful enough to motivate many of our bodily processes.

A truly relaxed body also exerts substantial downward pressure. A person weighing 150lb sinking into one heel-pad applies about 50lb per square inch, twice the pressure in the tires of many autos. This, and the air's own pressure, help to explain the power of a relaxed body in Tai Chi sport and combat. While this needn't be the main purpose of Tai Chi practice, it does illustrate the ability of a single human body to engender substantial energy without conscious effort.

An important influence has emerged from many years of daily Tai Chi practice, solo and otherwise. By daily I mean two to six hours, sometimes studying something brief or simple, and other times engaging in a variety of practices related to Tai Chi applications. The influence that I was slow to realize applies to every facet of the art. And it improves everything assuming basics are reasonably in place. It is simply repetition: of Mind intent, of bodily movement, and, crucially, of the link between them. If interested or in doubt, just do it again. But just as it takes several miles for a marathon runner to settle into rhythm, so at any one time it may take several sets (counting in eights, say) to begin feeling each intended move. This is no news to anyone able to step well through a complex form, or to someone adept in Tai Chi applications.

But you can't just think things into existence (except, perhaps, ideas). It is after all the will, need-intent, that transforms instinct or idea into action. And it is stories oft-told and deeds repeated that become effortlessly internalized. This common-sense applies, for example, to each breath followed in a simple standing posture. The same applies to releasing tension in rhythm with the breath. By applying relax to an in-breath and release to an out-breath, even this benefit can be doubled. Sooner or later the word transforms; there is a bodily change. Realization then emerges from deeper places into consciousness: Ah! if not Eureka! It happened in learning to walk; it can happen in Tai Chi practice.

Who knows how many parts there are to a solo form, or even if there are any parts? Only application of the principles is really important. There is no need for lists if you're engaging the instincts in emerging situations: the moves just keep coming. Any change or move in the solo form is an analog of the whole. In other words, a core description of any move will echo that of any other. Thus a complete form isn't all that useful unless each transition is correct, that is, functional. And this is a reason, perhaps, for the classic Oriental approach of learning exhaustively one move at a time. However, the wisdom of this path is readily apparent only after much practice. But it can be too difficult for beginners or other kinds of learners. For modern bodies, some Tai Chi Chuan is better than none.

But by treating each move in a complete way, such that it is repeated in a smooth cycle, time and technique will meld into an efficient learning curve. It is highly beneficial to repeat a simple arm movement. The falling arm in single Ward-off is allowed to float down and up, up and down, many times. Each direction is influenced by relaxation on the arm's **underside**, just as it is in a bubble rising or a raindrop falling. A wave-like motion through the arm, like a pennant in a breeze, reveals itself as a unit of movement. And by repeating an experience without goal (Cheng Man-ching: Don't be greedy), you distil a unit of movement from a sequence of events. The same principle and method apply to any component of movement in any limb.

These parts readily combine into a more complex whole. A rising arm, a falling arm, a weight-shift, a torso-turn, learned as components, can be overlaid and sequenced into Ward-off. The key is repeatability, adding one good move to another. That's why basics are so important. Why practice errors, however small? So one move learned is added to another move learned. Then the two moves are practiced as one until this more complex component is learned. Then the third, followed by one-plus-two-plus-three, and so on. Each component needs to be internalized for this to work. If you need to think about it, you're on the wrong track or not there yet. Eventually short and long sequences become joined until, surprise, there is no sequence. Clarity in practice-method emerges seamlessly from deep instinct, just as it does for each heart-beat, breath, secretion, and transformation that flows into the act of living.

So much for the many. This many are merely spokes in the greater wheel, so to speak. As learning progresses, practicing a complex system engenders a reduction in numbers. Many components transform into one organism. If numbers don't reduce, practice is off-track or short on principle. Then as they decrease, as the need for lists falls away like useless tension, perhaps it's natural to ponder how few there can be. A recurring question arises from an emerging Tai Chi body: What is the relationship between optimal and minimal? Clearly there is a handful of basics, like gravity, heat, rhythm, flow, straight, round. But what glues structure and energy in an elastic human body seems to be simply **economy**. Economy. Engaging the demanding environment of Nature, including other life-forms has brought many face-to-face with this simple proposition: that economy is singular yet universally useful.

It seems to be the gateway to both survival and grace in a human body. Yet stated as basics, engaging economy seems a dry set of rules: practice Tai Chi Chuan, no more no less; do nothing unnecessary; don't interfere with natural movement. Well, these are basics that need to be realized in acquiring a natural body, one that compares favorably with those of wild animals. A major advantage of sensing natural (or wild) fluid, elastic integration is that it feels so good. It is just like watching a nature program in your own body. Why not? Everyone can manifest grace. And all it entails is ridding bodily movement of useless distractions and destructive habits. These in turn are rendered redundant merely by inviting economy into what one does. It is the angular and awkward habits of too much and too little that interfere with a human's natural grace.

Nothing tests integration more than a prospect of terminal disintegration in life-or-death engagement. Such serious threats to life take many forms. Sickness, for example. A body already weakened or unprepared may succumb when a healthier, more united one may not. Starvation really brings one to contemplate what is essential to bodily survival, as does fasting to a lesser degree. Extreme climate has tested many to the limit of understanding conservation. And merely moving from one part of the earth to another via demanding terrain has spelled life or death to many.

Tai Chi Chuan's most trying tests originate in warfare. If you have survived life-threatening battles, you've probably learned something useful to apply to the battlefield of everyday life, so to speak. Self-preservation is another way of saying maintenance. It's a dynamic balance exercised by all viable organisms. Easy-going situations may be comfortable, and there's nothing wrong with that. When the going is more difficult, however, a body that has only ever been comfortable may not be the best instrument for continued well-being. When predators hunt, as is their prerogative, they tend to choose less robust quarry as their target for the next meal. This meal is not to satisfy casual whim, but is necessary to self-preservation in the hunters' lives, including dependents. They must be on their mettle, therefore, or there is no meal. Only about five to 10% of hunts are successful. Whatever the organism, it must sustain its faculties and its abilities throughout many forays. It must be fit because it is constantly being tested by the quarries' own self-preservation.

Tai Chi Chuan emerged from its jealously-guarded privacy because the core practices of this fighting art could address the problem of a population weakened by bad habits. A stronger nation was the aim, and more integrated people in better health was seen as its source. Occupation: farmer, official, laborer, or warrior, was not the issue. And Tai Chi Chuan was not chosen only for its martial qualities. Its ability to yield stronger, versatile humans applies to self-preservation in any circumstances.

Tai Chi practices had already been tested in combat, the worst possible conditions. Not for nothing was Yang Lu-chan known as invincible. Thus the graceful flow of Tai Chi movement had a severe counterpart in its ability to prevail in mortal combat. One has to do what needs to be done. The cold logic of this principle is, however, merely the counterpart of righteous preservation of life and limb. Even if you begin Tai Chi practice with the aim of kicking butt, by the time the necessary skills have been acquired, all of that initial urge will be long gone. The training is arduous and integrative, a foundation for true personal improvement.

Thus the economy implicit in four ounces defeating a thousand pounds is the result of relaxation, alignment, balance, sensitivity, and seamless adaptation to change. The strategy is to maintain the center, to self-preserve. When some invading energy seeks to impinge on this equilibrium, Tai Chi tactics redress the imbalance as it emerges. The energy is low, and the time short, such that the continued well-being of the person under attack is seamless. Four ounces is more than enough to deflect someone briefly, if the energy arrives as a pulse in the right place at the right time. These conditions of correctness, that is, efficacy, are engendered by training. Bear in mind that a four-ounce pulse moving rapidly and accelerating into a sensitive place is no small matter. Think of a smooth stone swinging on a rope, then add the energy of spin to the rock. The effect in Tai Chi application is of a twist-drill in hammer mode at about four beats/second.

Applying such knowledge is a matter of deep study, no less demanding than the acquisition of skills in, say, acupuncture. Furthermore, the receiving body is not static nor amenable to the technique. Thus Tai Chi technique is applied rapidly and accurately or it is ineffective, at least as a pulse. In time-scales other than immediate, Tai Chi practice applies its more yin qualities. While yielding and deflection can be invisibly fast, manipulation usually takes longer than pulses (though no longer than a series of pulses). But all maneuvers in Tai Chi Chuan, including deceptive ones, comprise the same principles of movement. Dealing with a series of moments is less fruitful and less secure than dealing with one. If you're stuck in the first moment there may be no second. So it is primarily important to maintain yin by releasing as soon as possible after a yang pulse. That's some undertaking at rates of several per second.

Therefore awareness is one thing, consciousness another. Thinking has no place nor time in applied Tai Chi Chuan. Conscious thought, however rapid, always lags instinctual intent. The thinking-mind and the exterior muscles occupy the same realm. That's one reason why intrinsic energy tends to be interrupted by physical force, however small. When the interior leads and the exterior follows, the result is usually smooth and favorable. It is also integrated and direct. Would you send a bullet down a dirty dented barrel? And even if you did, would a long or a short bullet have the better chance?

Economy, realized via the twin principles of alignment and relaxation, is the heart of Tai Chi Chuan. We might add that the context is righteous application. Practicing correct or effective solo form enhances human health and maintains it under whatever circumstances arise. Tai Chi Chuan is not a relaxing exercise or a martial art, it is both. There are many Tai

Chi games that serve both purposes equally. That is as it should be in a whole-body discipline of a complex organism.

Such propositions may sit uneasily in formally educated minds. This is just an example of the intellect being fooled by its own invention, external logic. Anyway, conscious thought is a process least useful for vital functions, a view common to practicers in many internal disciplines. There are special methods applying conscious energy to internal processes, but they lie outside the scope of this manual, and are unnecessary to progress. We just don't need to think about natural movement; other complex creatures don't, do they? We can instead apply our senses to the events of our practice. Allowing our attention to dwell at the center is something we sense. And there is no need to think about emptying the thinking-mind. Tai Chi practice will do that for us. Stealth, neutralization, and evasion are as useful within as they are in the external realm.

These considerations share common ground with an icon revered by many aspiring martial artists, that of the noble warrior. Do heroes aspire to nobility? Is there ever a time for such? Certainly not in the moment of deed. And anyway, a Tai Chi practicer realizes sooner or later that all notions, including nobility, are distant from the center. And that the lower dantien is a little low for such high thoughts. But any person or warrior may well realize the grace of true economy, and even sense pleasure in it.

Printed in the United States
125187LV00006B/140/A